Y0-AGW-844

4.95
Carolyn
Johnson
Oct 14-06

man
MANAGEMENT

over 350 ways to get the most from your man

THIS IS A CARLTON BOOK
Text, design and illustrations copyright © 2003
Carlton Books Limited
This edition published by Carlton Books Limited 2005
20 Mortimer Street, London W1T 3JW

This book is sold subject to the condition that it shall not, by
way of trade or otherwise, be lent, resold, hired out or otherwise
circulated without the publisher's prior written consent in any
form of cover or binding other than that in which it is published
and without a similar condition including this condition being
imposed upon the subsequent purchaser.

Material for this book has previously appeared under the titles
Over 100 Ways to Get a Man (Carlton, 2001*), Over 100 Things
Women Should Know About Men* (Carlton, 2002) and *Over 100
Ways to Leave Your Lover* (Carlton, 2002).

All rights reserved.
A CIP catalogue record for this book is available
from the British Library.

ISBN 1 84442 481 2

Printed and bound in Singapore

Executive Editor: Zia Mattocks
Design: DW Design
Copy Editors: Toira Leitch and Jane Donovan
Illustrator: Robert Loxton
Production Controller: Caroline Alberti

man
MANAGEMENT

over 350 ways to get the most from your man

LISA SUSSMAN

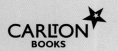

CARLTON
BOOKS

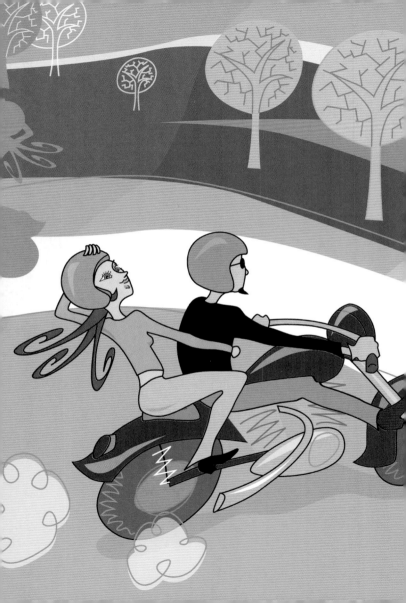

CONTENTS

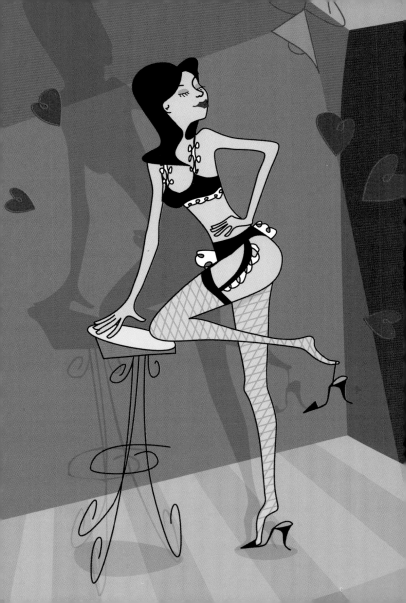

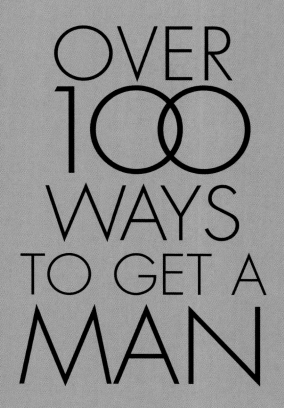

OVER
100
WAYS
TO GET A
MAN

When You Have Three Seconds

Studies confirm that the impression you make in the first **three seconds** is the lasting one. We make up our minds in an instant about how sexy we find the other person.

Here's what to do when you have just a few moments to grab his attention. Remember, though, while it's good to tune into your gut instincts, never put yourself in a vulnerable position with a stranger where you are on your own with him in a secluded place, and don't tell him your address.

ACCESSORIZE

Sometimes all it takes is the right prop to catch
a guy's eye.

Use the novel approach. Certain books
are guaranteed to put him in the mood
to chat. *Fever Pitch*, *Zen and the Art
of Motorcycle Maintenance* and *The
Hitchhiker's Guide to the Galaxy* are
all good guy-catchers.

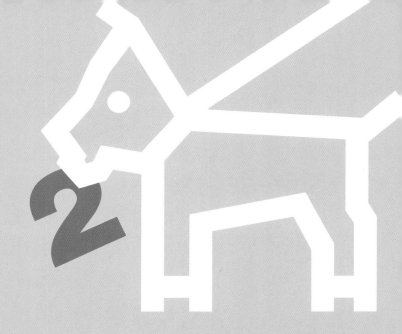

Men are often more comfortable talking about – and to – **big friendly dogs** than they are about approaching a woman. So take your pooch – or borrow one – for a leisurely walk in the park. Bring along a toy and throw it in the direction of an attractive prospect. Or (accidentally-on-purpose) hit him on the head with your ball. That's sure to get him talking.

Grab your camera (film optional). When you see someone you want to talk to, hold up the camera and say, 'Fromage!'

Go fly a kite. And don't be upset if you can't get yours airborne. Keep trying until you spot the guy you want to help you.

DOUBLE TAKES

Consider yourself warned: these five subtle, but totally sexifying beauty moves will inexplicably draw every man in the area directly towards you.

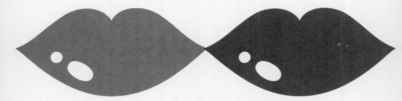

5 **Spellbind him** with lips he'll lust for. A berry shade whispers seductively, while a deep vibrant red shouts, 'Look at me!'

Tempt him to **touch you** by massaging baby oil into your skin. Go out and enjoy your new high TQ (touchability quotient) by 'accidentally' brushing your bare arm against a cute guy's biceps. Instead of apologizing, simply smile – silky seductive skin means never having to say you're sorry.

6

Captivate him with your **alluring cleavage**. While a push-up bra can make your bosom perk up, a subtle golden shimmer will make it stand out among the masses. For a stare-if-you-dare divide, smooth on a sparkling sheer liquid bronzer from collarbone to cleavage, concentrating some colour in between your breasts to create the illusion of a deep, lusty neckline.

7

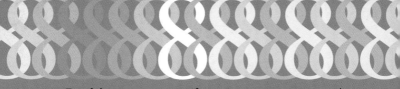

Eroticize your scent. If you want your scent to draw guys in like bees to honey, avoid the number one fragrance faux pas: perfume overload. Forgo heavy scents for a subtle citrus fragrance that he'll sneak up closer to sniff.

9

Tease him with lustrous locks. **Catch his eye** with the world's shiniest coif. Rinsing beaten egg whites into your head during your shower will add instant moisture, shine and bounce.

GIVE YOURSELF A MAKEOVER

Knock-'em-out beauty is within your control.

Get a facial. Studies have revealed that the one thing that's guaranteed to make his head do a 360-degree turn is smooth, shiny skin (glossy hair doesn't hurt either). It's a sign of high oestrogen levels and difficult-to-mimic signs of youthfulness and fertility.

Dye your hair blonde. Research has found that blondes are more likely to be seen as eye candy than people with darker colouring.

Get dolled up. When a New Mexico State University study recorded beauty preferences, it was found that the look that made his eyes pop is a high forehead, full lips, a short jaw, a small chin and nose, big eyes and knife-sharp cheekbones. In short, Barbie lives.

Do your abs. A University of Texas study suggests that men prefer a 0.7 waist-to-hip ratio (i.e., the hips are roughly a third larger than the waist), possibly because it broadcasts a female's health and readiness to breed. For the record, Cindy Crawford and Naomi Campbell inch in with a 0.69 ratio. But so does anyone with a 70-cm (28-in) waist and 100-cm (40-in) hips – which just happens to be 47 per cent of the UK female population.

SCENT HIM OUT

Smell is sexual chemistry in the most basic sense of the phrase. In a recent survey by the Fragrance Foundation, both men and women rated scent as an important aspect of sex appeal, giving odour an 8.4 rating on a scale of ten.

Follow your cycle. Researchers have established that a woman smells significantly different during ovulation – the time when she is most likely to become pregnant and therefore most needs to attract a mate – and that men are capable of sniffing out this change.

15 Use a **green-apple** scented lip gloss, then move in close. The scent has been found to work the limbic or sex part of the brain.

Stub out your cigarette. People who smoke are at a considerable disadvantage when it comes to smelling the subtle scents of sex. Smokers cover up their own natural scents, too, which puts others literally 'off the scent' – not to mention ash breath, yellow teeth and prematurely wrinkled skin. Bottom line: unless you're Bette Davis, lighting up cools his flame.

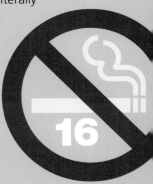

Douse yourself with lavender. Scientists have discovered that just a whiff of this fragrance can increase his penile blood-flow by 40 per cent, proving it to be quite the man-magnet. Other hot scent combos include **black liquorice and doughnuts**, and doughnuts and pumpkin pie.

Skip the perfume. Humans produce their own airborne, 'here I am, come and get me' aromatic signals to the opposite sex. These are known as pheromones. Just stroll past and spritz him.

Around the world, **sweat** is used as a love potion. An old Caribbean recipe reads: 'Prepare hamburger patty. Step in your own sweat. Cook. Serve to the person desired.'

FOLLOW YOUR INSTINCTS

There's more to animal magnetism than meets the eye. Scientists have found that it's not that men are suckers for good looks; rather, they're genetically programmed to seek out a certain KIND of looks.

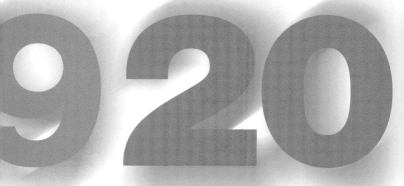

920

Stop dieting. Researchers at the University of Pennsylvania in Philadelphia showed pictures of female bodies ranging from almost skeletal to Rubenesque and found that it's not the men who plump for skinny women – it's the women. Biology dictates that women need a certain amount of body fat to produce hormones, periods and breasts (i.e. to produce offspring).

Go for an older guy – or **lie about your age**. According to a study of over 10,000 people in 37 countries, men are basically suckers for anyone younger than them (they equate youth with fertility).

According to the **symmetry theory** of physical attractiveness, callipers may be the only male-baiting accessory you need. It seems that humans, like most other species, show a strong preference for individuals who, when you draw a line down the centre of their body from their forehead to their toes, match up perfectly on the left and right sides. Studies have found that well-balanced babes have more – and better – sex than their lopsided counterparts. They're even more likely to have synchronized orgasms.

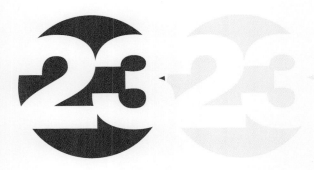

Look for your male twin. The reason why? Imprinting. People tend to be subconsciously attracted to replications of their parents. Hopefully they'll nurture you in the same way – only better. After years of trying to avoid becoming like Mum and Dad, we now look to date them.

Don't stand out. Studies show that from England to Australia and even a sprinkling of hunting/gathering tribes, the facial ideal of attractiveness tends to be very middle-of-the-road. It's thought to be a prehistoric instinct that the more average a person is, the less likely they are to carry nasty health problems that will end up infecting the gene line.

24

Go pulling just before your period when your **oestrogen levels** surge. This is the Marilyn Monroe of hormones. It makes you feel finger-licking desirable and more likely to be chatted up.

25

CREATE CHEMISTRY

You can't score if you're not playing the field.
Ninety per cent of life is about showing up in the
first place. Go out to places with signs of life –
intelligent or otherwise – and use these tricks.

26

Dress like you're a success. When
researchers showed photographs
to a group of men of one particular
woman, either dressed comfortably
or wearing a business suit, the men
rated the nicely dressed version to
be much more appealing, without
realizing it was the same woman.
Talk about a power suit!

Make the first move. Ninety-five per cent of men polled said they would love to be approached by a woman.

27@95%

A New England centre for the Study of the Family discovered that **WHERE** you meet someone for the first time can strongly influence attraction. For instance, when men met a woman in the gym, they thought she was sexy and healthy-looking. But when they ran into the same woman at the pub, they rated her as unattractive.

28

Get in his **line of vision** so he notices you. Ninety-nine per cent of attracting a guy's attention is about getting him to see you in the first place.

Give up. That's right, forget about finding a date. Instead, start finding out what it is you love to do and what (besides the entire male species) fascinates and enthralls you most. When you stop waiting around for a guy to change your life, Mr Wonderful is most likely to show up. Ironic, huh?

If you **go out** with a group of friends or even just one girlfriend, make sure you separate off from them so that you appear to be more approachable. No man wants to be rejected in front of a group of women, and he may well feel he cannot approach you when you are 'protected' by a herd of other women!

31

HEAD MOVES TO MAKE
HIM NOTICE YOU

Sometimes all he needs is a nod in the right direction.

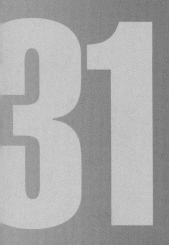

32

Toss your head. This is the classic attention-grabber. Flip your head back so your face tilts upwards. The movement attracts his eye as your face catches the light. It means: 'Hi, look at me' (usually used at the same time as tip 36 below).

33 Let him know you care with a **flip of the hair**. Raise one hand and push your fingers through your hair. This can be done once, slowly and thoughtfully, or in short spurts, pulling your hair back and drawing attention to your face. He'll think you're gorgeous and come your way. Follow this up with tip 35.

34 The head **nod** is usually done when you're passing almost nose-to-nose. Nod your head gently backwards and forwards until you're communicating by moving together in a gentle sway. It's a quick way to tell him, 'Come with me, I'm more than interested.'

35 The Eyebrow Flash is the first of what psychologists call 'the looks'. Raise both eyebrows in an exaggerated gesture, follow by lowering your eyes quickly to establish eye contact momentarily. As the eyebrows rise to their peak, the eyeballs are exposed because the eyelids lift and the muscles around the eyes stretch, allowing more light onto the surface of the eyes. This makes them appear large and bright, and very attractive. It's a genetically programmed classic come-on.

36 Tilt your head to one side and smile. You trigger a subtle sexual arousal in him by revealing a portion of your neck – even though the gesture suggests a certain demureness. (Think of Princess Di's famous head tilt and smile.) The more you tilt your head, the more you're showing your interest. Throw some lip-licking and side-glancing into the mix (see tips 60 and 63) and you'll have him on his knees.

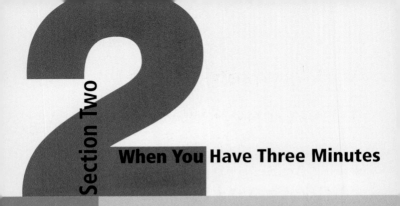

2

When You Have Three Minutes

Your next move is the one that has the
power to reduce a man to a trembling
wreck. It's not beauty or even big breasts
that attract men – it's knowing how
to play the game. Make no mistake –
flirting works. There's no better way
to grab and hold a man's attention.

Here are some sexy follow-up strategies
for when you have a few more minutes
on your side. Beware: these moves are
guaranteed to turn even the biggest
stud into a love-struck puppy.

WORK YOUR BODY

These body moves are sure to entice him.

Crossing your arms is a natural instinctive response
when you're feeling vulnerable. The problem is,
it signals DO NOT APPROACH. To avoid doing this,
put one hand in your pocket, on your hip or on the
arm of a chair. Or hold something like a drink or
a pen (useful for exchanging phone numbers).

Working out is a great way to get male attention – not because you might meet guys at the gym (although you probably will), but because you will love the way a strong healthy body feels when you have the energy and ability to do anything. When you're comfortable with yourself, you inevitably come across as being more confident, sexy and fun.

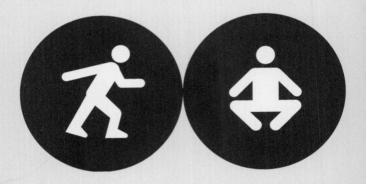

Practise a sexy walk. Stand up straight, take a stride about one and a half times the length of your foot. This is the distance men are biologically fine-tuned to read as a sign of health and fertility, making you a hot prospect for passing on their genes. **39**

When you **slide onto a bar stool**, sit with your legs crossed at the knee in what's called the Leg Twine. To wrap him around your little toe, languidly stroke your calf and let your shoe fall partly off.

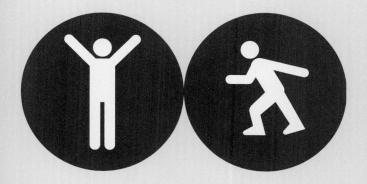

Get the same effect from a distance by **crossing your legs** so they point towards a nearby cutie, showing that you'd like to enter his personal space (about 0.9 m/3 ft, according to studies).

NO-TOUCH SEDUCTION

Here's how to get a man to approach you without even lifting a finger.

Get a flushed face by thinking of something sexy or embarrassing. It's a signal to him that you're attracted to him.

Guys are suckers for long tresses. So entwine him in **your locks** by running your fingers through your hair and tossing it in his direction.

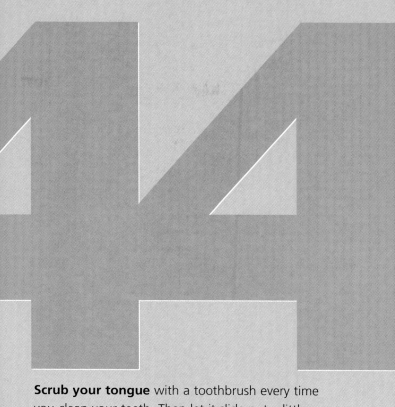

Scrub your tongue with a toothbrush every time you clean your teeth. Then let it slide out a little when your target is near. A healthy pink tongue is a visual turn-on for him.

Regular, **moderate exercise** alters
metabolic rates and hormone levels, which often
results in a greater sense of wellbeing and energy,
an aura of confidence and an increased level of
sexual desire – all powerful honey attractants.

When we first notice someone, we spend about
three seconds scanning their face, flicking our
eyes backwards and forwards between the other
person's eyes, then moving down to the mouth
and finishing off with a few broader sweeps that
take in the hair. Extending the scan to four-and-a-
half seconds will create strong emotions in him.

47

Buy time with a smile. Studies have found that when you smile at someone, they take a longer look because they are made to feel at ease.

HOW TO GET A MAN'S ATTENTION – ANYWHERE, ANYTIME

Now you've spotted him, here are some new, improved ways to catch his eye, start a conversation and keep it going.

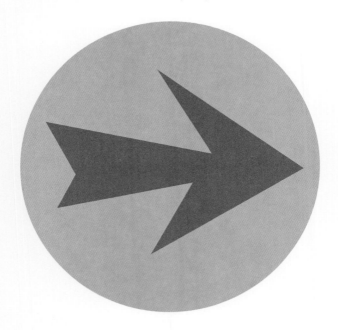

ON THE STREET: Ask for directions – even if you live in the neighbourhood.

WHAT YOU SHOULD SAY: 'Excuse me,' which should then, in a millisecond, tell you how receptive he's going to be to you. If he seems to welcome the intrusion, ask the whereabouts of a shop, restaurant or bar.

WHY THIS WILL WORK: Men love to be helpful (and act like know-it-alls).

POSSIBLE NEXT MOVE: After he gives you the instructions, say, 'I should write this down.' At that point, you should pull out a pen and paper and scribble down the directions. This will prolong the encounter, and if he's interested, he'll wait. If a prolonged conversation starts, since you already have your pen and paper out, you can ask for his number.

AT A SUPERMARKET: Ask him a practical question and allow him the chance to help you out. Use the many hidden mysteries of the supermarket as a jumping-off point.

WHAT YOU SHOULD SAY: 'Do you know where they keep the crisps?' Then follow him around the aisles to find them. Or say, 'Can you reach that roll of paper towels?' or 'Can you believe how much this costs?' Or point out some snack choice in his cart (you'll have lots to choose from!) and say, 'Excuse me, but is that good? I'm supposed to bring something to a party later.'

WHY THIS WILL WORK: A direct question is always answerable and if he rebuffs you, you can always save face by asking the very next passer-by the same question (so your target ends up looking like a rude people-phobe).

POSSIBLE NEXT MOVE: More questions: 'I don't shop here that often. Is it always this crowded?' This is one step away from saying, as ironically as possible, 'So, do you come here often?' It leads to talk of his shopping schedule, which gives you information on his lifestyle (as does the contents of his cart), which can open the door to a million other topics of conversation.

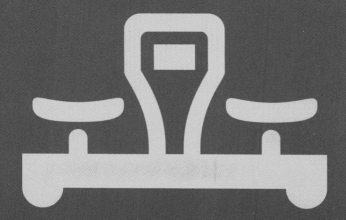

50

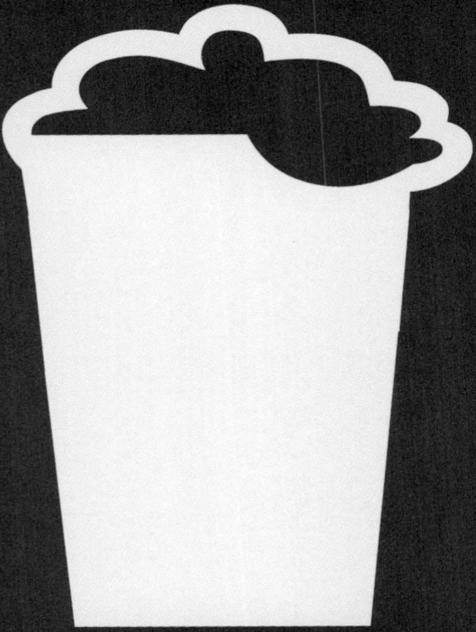

IN A BAR: Stand near him, sip your drink and look deeply perturbed.

WHAT YOU SHOULD SAY: 'I might be going crazy, but does my drink taste soapy to you?' Hold out your glass to him. It doesn't matter if he takes you up on your offer to taste it. You've made the opening to say, 'I'm going to order another. Can I get you something?'

WHY THIS WILL WORK: It has nothing to do with talking about him, about you, or why you're both in the bar.

POSSIBLE NEXT MOVE: If he accepts your offer of a drink, comment on his beverage of choice. He wants a Bud? Say, 'Would you believe I tried draft for the first time recently,' which will launch a conversation about draft versus bottled. If he gets a cocktail, ask about the origin of its name, 'Who do you think Tom Collins was anyway?'

AT THE LAUNDRY: While fussing with a machine, surreptitiously drop a coin in such a way that it goes between the machines. Loudly express your frustration and attempt to pull the machines apart.

WHAT YOU SHOULD SAY: 'Oh no. I've lost so much money this way! I'll bet there's a fortune between these machines.'

WHY THIS WILL WORK: You've provided a conversation opener, and you've given him the opportunity to engage in a complaint-fest over the vagaries of doing your laundry. He might even figure out a way to help you get your money back.

POSSIBLE NEXT MOVE: Once you've been talking (or you're joined in an effort to move the washer), ask him where he lives. (It must be nearby.) Then you can discuss the neighbourhood, the building, favourite sports and so on.

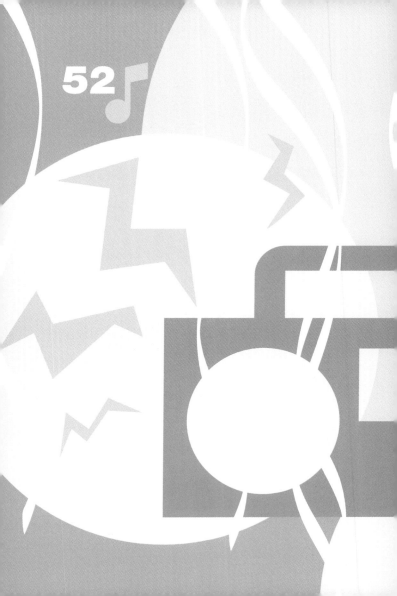

AT A PARTY: Look over and smile. Smile in a big, appreciative way. Smile as if there's a caption over your head that reads, 'I'm having a great time and I'm so glad to see you.'

WHAT YOU SHOULD SAY: After edging towards him over the course of 15 minutes, say, 'Hello.' Introduce yourself. Be a human being about it, it's a party, after all. You're supposed to go to them to meet people and mingle, so you shouldn't be too embarrassed to actually attempt to do so.

WHY THIS WILL WORK: Everyone's awkward at a party and he'll be thrilled to see a friendly, happy face.

POSSIBLE NEXT MOVE: After 'Hello,' traditional follow-ups are, 'What brings you here?' or 'What's going on?' If he has any social skills at all, conversation should ensue. Once you've been talking for a while (say, half an hour), you can always make the 'It's pretty noisy in here' or 'It looks as though people are leaving' observation and casually suggest moving on to another venue, like a place to get coffee.

AT A CLUB: Have fun on the dance floor AND look like you are, too. Often, when you dance, you're so caught up with what you look like or who's checking you out that you forget to relax and enjoy yourself. Then exit the floor, get a big glass of water and stand near the guy you're interested in.

WHAT YOU SHOULD SAY: 'I was wondering what the view was like from over here, and, please, tell me that I look pretentious/silly/ embarrassing on the dance floor!'

WHY THIS WILL WORK: A woman who doesn't take herself too seriously on a dance floor looks approachable.

POSSIBLE NEXT MOVE: He'll assure you that you dance divinely. Should mutual attraction happen, you could then say, 'Do you dance? Or do you come here just for the music?' If he wants to dance (and this is a huge deal for lots of men), he'll take the hint and ask you. If not, don't ask him, since his refusal could make for an awkward moment. And yes, we could ponder on why some guys go to clubs when they don't dance, but it's still a good place to meet women, right?

53

ORAL PLEASURES

How to sweet-talk him with pick-up lines guaranteed to work.

A University of Louisiana study found that the following phrases will perk up his ears (and other organs):

- 'Hi.' (97 per cent success rate)

- 'Would you like another beer?' (91 per cent success rate)

- Introducing yourself (88 per cent success rate)

- Put your sweater or jacket down on the bar and say, 'Can you do me a massive favour and watch this for a second? I have to run to the ladies' room.' (85 per cent success rate)

- 'I feel a little embarrassed about this, but I'd like to meet you.' (82 per cent success rate)

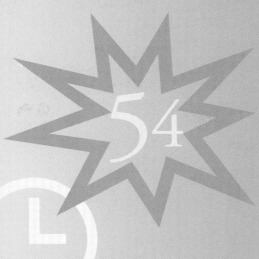

- Touch his watch and ask, 'Do you have the time?' (81 per cent success rate)

- Instead of asking him what he does, ask him what he enjoys doing (78 per cent success rate)

- If you're at a party, walk up and say, 'Could I talk to you for a couple of minutes? There's someone I'm trying to avoid.' (76 per cent success rate)

- 'What do you think of the band/food/movie?' (70 per cent success rate)

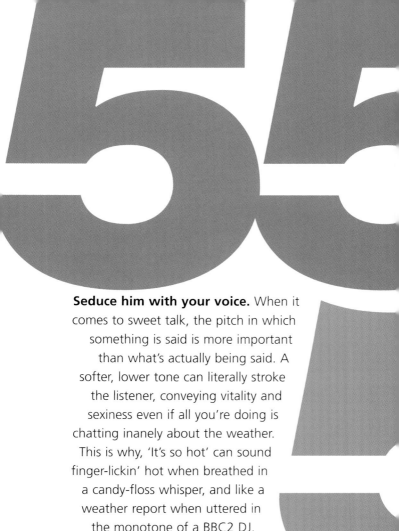

Seduce him with your voice. When it comes to sweet talk, the pitch in which something is said is more important than what's actually being said. A softer, lower tone can literally stroke the listener, conveying vitality and sexiness even if all you're doing is chatting inanely about the weather. This is why, 'It's so hot' can sound finger-lickin' hot when breathed in a candy-floss whisper, and like a weather report when uttered in the monotone of a BBC2 DJ.

Tell him a secret. Disclosure gets him on your side. Lean in and tell him something personal – even if it's whether or not you're happy in your job. Men are attracted to that comfortable feeling of safety, so this makes it easier for him to share as well. But don't reveal too much about yourself (see tip 81 for why).

When You Have 30 Minutes

Flirting is the most subtle form of man-I-pul(ation) there is. But playing hard to get is an art form that takes practice. Successful flirting is all about telling the truth about yourself but not giving the whole game away.

Here are some man-baiting tactics for when you're pubbing or clubbing, or when you're at a party. And if you think they're too outrageous for you, remember: if there were no women out there who made the first move, most men would still be virgins.

STRUT YOUR STUFF

Being aggressive with a stranger is a no-lose situation. If he's already noticed you, then he's thrilled; if he hasn't, then you're only making yourself less invisible to him. These no-holds-barred moves will make him look twice (and ask for your number).

It may seem polite to leave a little room between you and the guy you're interested in, but extreme flirting is no place for politeness! **Lean in towards him** to give him the impression that you want to exclude everyone else in the world.

57

58

Go for the kill by sidling up next to him and letting him **feel your heat**. Stand so close that you're almost touching him. When you step into his personal space, he interprets it as an immediate sexual invitation. If you stand close enough to a man for him to kiss you, he'll probably try.

Stroking your lower neck can cause your nipples to become firm. He'll happily take things from there.

60

Lick your lips when you look at him. Wet lips seem to simulate vaginal lubrication, signalling that he makes you horny.

Bump into him at the bar. Then, instead of saying, 'Excuse me,' put your hand on his back. Use gentle pressure, as if he were already your lover. When he looks to see who's behind him, say 'I'm sorry, I was just trying to get past.' Then flash him an innocent smile and move on. Guaranteed he'll be right on your trail.

62

Read HIS body moves:
- He chews faster
- His lips part slightly as he makes eye contact
- He touches his hair
- He touches his face more, stroking his cheeks, ears or neck
- He unconsciously (we hope) points at his genitals

STARE HIM DOWN

Your eyes are 18 times more sensitive than your ears. Use them to captivate him.

The first rule men learn about picking up women is not to make an approach before they get the all-clear. One glance means a possible, 'Yes'. Two glances means, 'Come over'. Three glances and you're telling him, **'What's taking you so long?'**

Holding his gaze for two seconds is the magic number – any shorter than this and he can't be sure you're interested; any longer and he might call the cops!

Try the Two-Eyed Wink. A slower version of a normal blink, with all the playfulness (and none of the cheese factor) of a regular wink. Glance his way, then blink slowly and smile. Wait for him to smile in response, then look away again.

65

6

Try smiling with just your eyes.

7

If you're shy, gaze at his **'third eye'** – the space between the eyebrows. He won't suspect a thing, but he will feel as though you are looking straight into his eyes.

68

Stay in the dark. Dilated pupils send out smouldering 'Notice me' messages, even if the distension is simply the result of bad lighting.

69

Short-sighted women have a peculiar attraction for many men, possibly because their unfocused gaze seems attentive. If you wear glasses, you can get the same effect by taking them off.

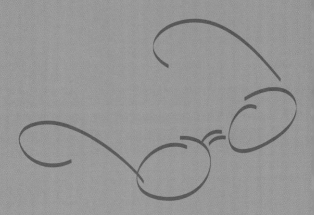

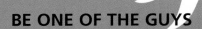

BE ONE OF THE GUYS

Adopting certain guy-like behaviour will make him
feel more comfortable about approaching you.

70 Know when the **hunting season** is. After
scrutinizing birth records from around the
world, German researchers concluded that
there's a definite human mating season
during the months when the sun shines
for about 12 hours per day and the
temperature hovers between 10 and 21
degrees C (50 and 70 degrees F). This
means, biologically, you're more likely
to look good to the opposite sex during
these times of the year.

71

Hang out with just the guys: it makes other guys wonder why you're such a man magnet, and all that testosterone sends your flirty side soaring.

Drink beer out of a bottle. It tells him that you're down-to-earth and unpretentious, and he can be himself around you. (And that's not to mention the obviously erotic gesture of wrapping your lips around a long cylindrical object.) Cheers!

72

Ignore him. After giving him the once-over, pretend that watching paint dry would be more interesting than looking at him. It seems that while playing hard to get may be bad news for your reputation, it'll do wonders for your social calendar. Men are more often attracted to someone they have to 'chase' than someone who may be just as pretty, but more readily available. Apparently, having an urge frustrated can intensify the feeling of need, making him interpret it as must-have desire.

Don't leave until **closing time**. As the night wears on, magically, you become better-looking. In a study of singles-bar patrons, as closing time neared, people's judgement of a person's attractiveness increases. The reason: a psychological mechanism sensitive to shrinking opportunities. As the mating pool thins, what's left looks better and better. Of course, the next morning things may seem different!

You've attracted him enough to snag a first date. Now, make him yours.

All a man really wants to know is that you like him. The trouble is, some women send out weaker signals than a cell phone submerged in water to let a man know they're interested. And if he thinks you're not into him, he'll want out of there. So, here's all you need to know to make him know that he is, without doubt, making your heart go flip-flop – without being TOO obvious about it.

DRESS FOR SEXCESS

Stylish moves that will guarantee he'll be ga-ga for good.

75

Wear something **touch-worthy**. A teasing hint of faux fur, a flirty feathered bracelet or anything else that's temptingly tactile can serve as a must-feel attention 'grab-her'. It'll catch his eye and make him want to stroke you.

Go au naturel. Using highly scented soaps and perfumes can interfere with his ability to detect your female scent, making him less likely to get turned on to you.

Get your accessories right. A poll by the University of California-Los Angeles found that guys regard a woman who accessorizes as a woman who cares about sex. The five top sexy adornments are:
* Thumb and toe rings
* Charm bracelet
* Red cars
* Red lipstick
* Black stockings

The colour of your clothes speaks volumes about you. Hot hues, especially scarlet, are linked with sexuality. In a study from Loyola University, Louisiana, both men and women rated red the most alluring shade, followed by dark blue, violet, black and yellow (virginal white didn't even get a look-in). Breathing and heart rates rise in the presence of strong red colours, so bright red actually makes him **physically aroused**.

Borrow his mum's clothes. The more you look like his mother or sister, the better your chances. It seems that after years of trying to avoid becoming like Mum and Dad, we now look to date them. A study from Rutgers University, New Jersey, found that people subconsciously tend to be attracted to replications of their parents or siblings in order to heal the emotional and psychological damage we all experience to some degree in childhood.

79

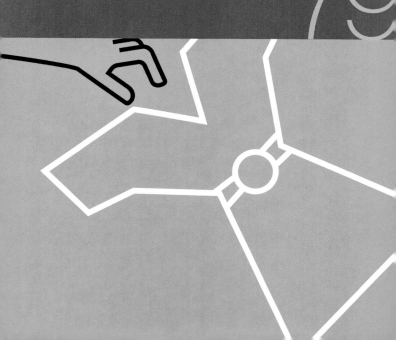

Call to him using a 'genital echo'. According to anything-that-moves watcher Desmond Morris, this alluring term covers all body parts with a passing resemblance to the genitals – in other words, a visual sexual double entendre. The belly button is one example, fingers another. (You figure out the matching genitals.) But the Big Mama of the pack is the mouth, which is thought to be a dead ringer for the vagina. In the same way as the inner labia of the vagina becomes bright red with engorged blood just prior to orgasm, our lips also become redder when we're turned on. Smearing your lips with red lipstick will send out an extra, 'I'm on the brink of ecstasy' announcement.

Wear a (figurative) **mask**. A little mystery is essential to infatuation. People almost never become captivated by someone they know well, as an Archives of Sexual Behaviour study on Israeli kibbutz marriages clearly illustrates. It was found that out of 2,769 marriages, none occurred between men and women who had actually grown up together on the kibbutz. And the reason for this? The easy familiarity of having spent their whole lives together was unconsciously translated into a chaste sibling bond instead of a passionate sexual one.

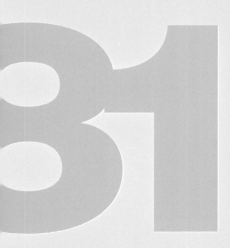

Show (off) some leg by hitching your skirt up slightly as you sit down. Or slip on a pair of high-heeled shoes, which enhances the length and shape of your **lower limbs**. This part of your body exerts an enormous sexual pull for some males. For many men, a long-legged look is dazzling, the reason being that the lengthening of the limbs is a feature of sexual maturity.

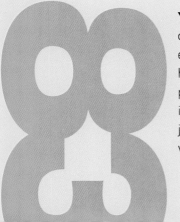

Your bottom sends out an unmistakable erotic message. Make him want to give it a pinch by wrapping it in a pair of tight-fitting jeans. You'll look like a voluptuous sex goddess.

GET HAPPY

Your mouth gives away your mood.
Make yours blissful ...

Smile only when you really mean it. A tight jaw
and top lip will seem false and make your face look
tension-filled and lopsided. The trick is to learn to
relax your face. Practise by scrunching up all your
facial muscles as tight as you possibly can for five
seconds and then release them. Do this five times,
then massage your temples.

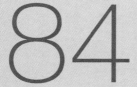

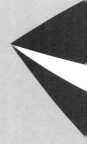

85

Bare your teeth: both men and women tend to give open smiles when they're sexually aroused.

86

Bite your lower lip as you smile. This is a very provocative move that will make him want to lean over and give you a long, lingering smooch.

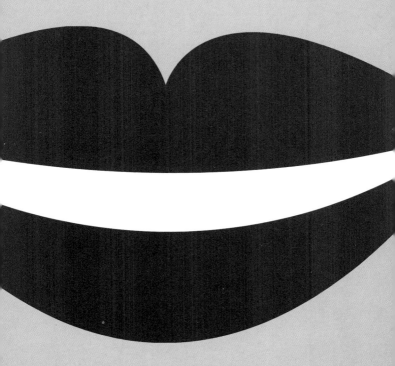

Smile with your mouth and eyes: this is the most friendly 'I'm-nice-to-know' smile there is. Think happy thoughts to get your face to light up. Adding a little laughter to the mix will put your body in a state of arousal similar to when you are sexually turned on and will make you seem more alluring.

Part your lips slightly when you smile. It'll make you seem alert, expressive and responsive. Susan Sprecher, PhD, professor of Sociology at Illinois University, conducted a cross-cultural survey of 1,667 men and women in the USA, Japan and Russia to find out what people look for in a mate. In all three countries, animation was a bigger draw than looks when it came to what made him want to get to know you better.

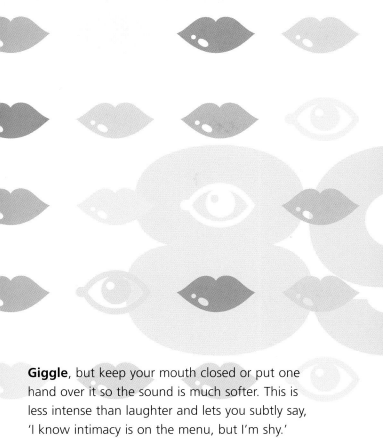

Giggle, but keep your mouth closed or put one hand over it so the sound is much softer. This is less intense than laughter and lets you subtly say, 'I know intimacy is on the menu, but I'm shy.'

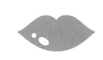

SAY IT WITH YOUR BODY

Try some of the body moves that will make him feel at ease and connected with you.

90

When you greet him, give off a sensual and **warm aura** when you're standing, simply by resting on one foot more than the other, letting your hip jut out a bit with your hands on the small of your back.

As you talk with him, point your knees, feet, hands, shoulders or whole body **towards him** – it's a subtle way of saying that you aren't complete strangers anymore.

Women, more than men, shrink into their spaces by subconsciously tightening their bodies. To avoid this, open your body to him. **Open your hands** instead of clenching them into fists. Don't fold them in a tight hand grasp; tent the fingertips instead, and rather than sitting with your hands tightly folded, drape them loosely over the arms of the chair. Bonus: the open body represents sexy power (a closed body symbolizes weakness, insecurity or hostility).

92

Affectionate touching tells a guy that you like him and that you wouldn't mind touching him more in private. If he says something witty, squeeze his forearm gently and laugh. If you want to go to the ladies' room, put your hand on his shoulder and say, 'I'll be right back.'

Copy him. When two people become captivated with each other, they begin to subtly and unconsciously mimic each other's postures and gestures within five to fifty seconds. Eventually, even breathing and heartbeats become synchronized. Called 'mirroring', it's a learned habit left over from infancy when the newborn mimics its body movements with the rhythmic patterns of whatever voice is speaking to it. You can consciously use mirroring to lure him in by deliberately echoing his movements. But keep it down to less than five gestures or he's going to feel stalked. (If he changes movements every time you start copying him, don't expect him to call you again.)

Sitting up with good, yet relaxed posture shows that you're having a good time and are interested in what he has to say.

Nod as he talks to show you're paying attention, but don't do it so much that you look as if your neck is on a spring, or you will end up putting a wall between you and your date. (It's the equivalent of crossing your arms.)

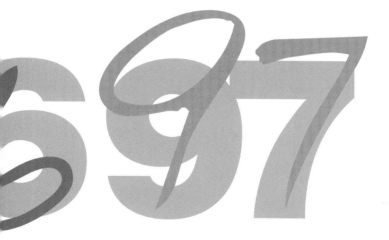

Use your body as well as your hands to express
what you mean. When you talk with your whole
body, you say,
**'I'm animated,
I'm interested,
I'm interesting.'**

Enchant him, tempt him, tease him. Any guy will tell you that it's the little gestures that achieve BIG results.

Best of all, when you have time on your hands, you can s-l-o-w-l-y blaze a sizzling impression on his radar. Check out these can't-resist-you tricks and dazzle the man you desire. Use them on him and in no time at all, he'll be drawn to you like a moth to a flame.

UNEXPECTED APHRODISIACS

Not-so-obvious ploys will make him stick around.

98

Hum 'Ode to Joy'. An Indiana University study of 239 students reveals that our musical tastes can influence how hot we think someone is, and men are more attracted to women with a taste for classical music (a man's desirability is amplified by a passion for heavy metal). They're still trying to work out why, but in the meantime, pump up the volume!

99

Eat raw mushrooms: the odour is reminiscent of sex. Or just eat in front of him, period. A New York University survey discovered that most guys think that a woman who picks at her food is a total turn-off (not to mention scary – it's no secret that the most mild-mannered person will turn into an irritable monster when they are food-deprived). Having a healthy appetite makes them think that you are going to be a sensuous lover.

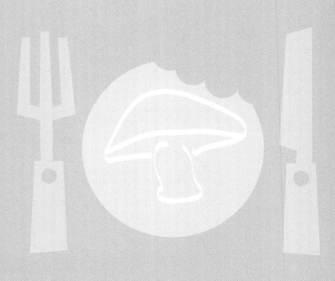

Practise listening. Believe it or not, just being attentive can be a turn-on for the object of your desire. Studies by language psychologist Deborah Tannen have found that women tend to interrupt more than men, making guys feel like they're not really being listened to. Keeping a little bit silent while you consider what he's saying will make you stand out because you're listening to him. And that will make him want to continue the conversation – over dinner, perhaps?

Scare yourselves sexy. Invite the object of your desire to a horror movie or for a ride on a roller-coaster. A Canadian study found that there's evidence that emotional arousal, including experiences that involve fear, triggers off sexual attraction. Research subjects who were either warned of imminent electric shock, scared to death on high, wobbly bridges or told of grotesque mutilations all tested higher for intensity of romantic passion. So did those who ran on the spot for two minutes, were severely embarrassed, or listened to a Steve Martin comedy routine.

FLIRTY FOREPLAY

Reduce an otherwise evolved man to a drooling, panting fool with these seductive gestures.

OnehundredandtwoOnehunddandtwoOnehundredandtu

Say his name to fan the flame. Called 'anchoring', the technique of saying his name three times while talking to him will connect him to you. Strengthen the bond between you physically by lightly touching his arm or hand when you repeat his moniker.

Use a nickname. According to a study by University of California-Los Angeles psychologist Albert Mehrabian, PhD, giving him your own private handle is a quick shortcut to making him feel up-close-and-personal with you.

PUMP UP THE PASSION

The sweet art of seduction is learning how to say, 'Come and get me' without making him feel stalked.

Check out the **material at work**. Most people select a job based on such factors as salary, status and enjoyment. But according to a study of 3,000 singles conducted by Pennsylvania State researchers, about 10 per cent of all love affairs begin between people who meet each other on the job (plus your love affair will have staying power). In another, more recent survey conducted by several temp agencies, about 2,000 career women claimed that a romance between colleagues is four times more likely to last than an affair between people who meet outside the workplace.

Pay a lot of **attention to his friends**. This triggers off a sense of rivalry in the guy you're after, forcing him to find a way into the conversation and exclude his buddy (never underestimate the competitiveness between men).

Along the same lines, **get a fake date**. If you know a great-looking male friend, by all means show him off. According to research on jealousy conducted by psychologist David Buss, PhD, there are few things more attractive to a man than the fact that other men are attracted to you. In one study, when people were asked to judge women based on photographs of them with 'spouses' of differing attractiveness, unattractive women paired off with good-looking men were routinely rated most favourably in terms of status.

107

Compete with him. Challenge him to a game of tennis and bust his balls. According to a study by John Jay College of Criminal Justice, women who don't hold back their killer instinct are seen as more attractive than those who act in a more demure fashion.

Cast a spell over him by throwing pink rose petals (they'll make him want to have sex) and fresh orange peel (for enticement) in your handbag or pocket. Lighting a pink candle before meeting up with him and visualizing how you want him to see you (as a sexy vixen, of course) will also influence his attitude.

108

GRAB HOLD OF HIM

Ways to touch him to let him know
you want him – NOW!

109

If you like him and you know it, **clap your hands**.
The truth is, we're more likely to be attracted to
someone who is obviously attracted to us. This give-
and-take element was confirmed in a University of
California study of passion influences, where the
perception of being liked ranked just as high as
the presence of sex appeal in the potential partner.

Flex and he'll think sex. Gestures exposing vulnerable areas such as the underside of your arms, sometimes while fondling a glass or keys, or running a fingertip along the arm of a table tell a man you are ready to expose yourself to him.

Remind him of what's **beneath your clothes**. Dangle a shoe off your bare toe or let the sleeve of your top slip off your shoulder so you're just a little more bare than he expects. One of the greatest turn-ons of all is imagining the parts of another person's body that you can't see. Showing him a little skin, even if it's not the most risqué spot, will be a hint of things to come ... if he plays his cards right.

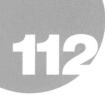

112

Scientists have observed that people tend to clasp their hands behind their head, elbows pointed skywards and armpits wafting outwards when they want to send out an arousal signal. It's a way of saying, 'Look at me. Listen to me. Smell me. **I'm sexy**.' (And who's going to argue with a couple of loaded armpits?)

Give him a little smooch. A Georgia Tech University study revealed that the sebaceous glands found all over the body act as a sort of bonding agent. When two people ingest each other's sebum, usually through a kiss, they become 'addicted' to each other's chemicals, making them want to couple up to maintain the warm, cuddly feelings all the time.

113

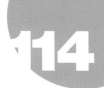

Give him an orgasm. A University of Manchester study indicates that when a person collapses in a joyful heap of contractual ripples, their brain levels of oxytocin, a sort of hormonal superglue, rise, making them feel more attracted and attached to their lover. Unfortunately, it doesn't work the other way around – the researchers found that the degree of romantic attachment had no effect on orgasm.

Caressing his head and face will have a similar effect to the above (but it isn't as much fun!).

Leave him guessing. Firmly clasp both your arms around his waist for no more than a few seconds. Then leave him to work out whether that embrace was 'sisterly' or not.

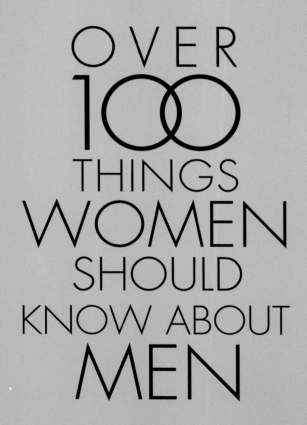

his **brain**

If you're anything like the average female, you sometimes have doubts about what planet men come from: Is he for real? Do all guys act this way? What is he THINKING?

Even though men and women both spend nine months in the womb, have 26 vertebrae in our spines and the same neurochemical pathways in our brains, we spend most of our years without any real understanding of what's actually going on in the other's brain.

Well, you can stop head-scratching (and ruining your 'do). Here's your field guide to the male species. This should settle once and for all why someone who pees differently is so different in every other way as well.

Caution: Don't read the following while eating. This unparalleled peek into the male mind may just make your jaw drop.

WHY CAN'T A MAN BE MORE LIKE A WOMAN?

Proof that Mother Nature favours her own sex.

Blahblahblah commitment. Blahblahblah cuddling. Blahblahblah seat up. This is what he hears when you talk. Evolutionary studies have found that the male hearing system isn't as fine-tuned as the female's (something to do with meat hunting being more important than baby nurturing). Hence, cut him some slack when he says he didn't hear you. He probably didn't.

Men and women don't use their brains in the same way. In general, men can only use either their left-brain language skills or their right-brain problem-solving skills, while women can use both at the same time. Which means that if he's talking, he's not thinking and if he's thinking, he's not talking.

From about age 12 to age 30, all men can think about is getting sex. That's because they're biologically driven to spread genes to as many babes as possible to ensure the survival of their DNA. Explaining why men are also so easy.

Why does he leave the toilet seat up, practically guaranteeing you'll find yourself hip-deep in toilet water at 3 am? It's all about power, say psychologists who study this sort of thing. It's his way of saying, 'Why is what you want more important than what I want?' (Er, because what a woman wants is more logical, perhaps?)

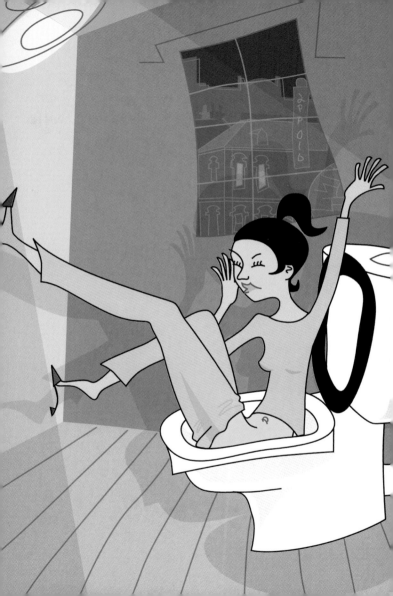

On the same theme, **his sheets are grimy, not because he has a male 'gross' gene, but because of biology.** Men have a weaker sense of smell and their skin isn't as sensitive as women's. So they aren't likely to notice (until live things are thriving) that they're snoozing on stinky sheets.

The average male is potty-trained by the age of three. So what's with the puddle on the floor? It turns out that peeing straight isn't as easy as it looks. The penis is a dual-purpose machine and many things – including sex – can create a blockage in the pipeline. And drips around the toilet.

It seems he has a scientific excuse for being lousy at figuring out how you feel. A Southern Methodist University found that **men rely on physical sensations, such as a racing heart or clammy hands, to clock moods, while women use visual factors like facial expressions to understand emotions.** Which means that if you're looking for sympathy from him, hand him a stethoscope.

The Y-chromosome set's rabid channel surfing could have something to do with brain degeneration. According to a study conducted at the University of Pennsylvania Medical Center, **men lose brain tissue three times faster than women,** with some of the largest losses in the parts that control attention span (explaining why he doesn't remember your anniversary, even after you've reminded him 623 times).

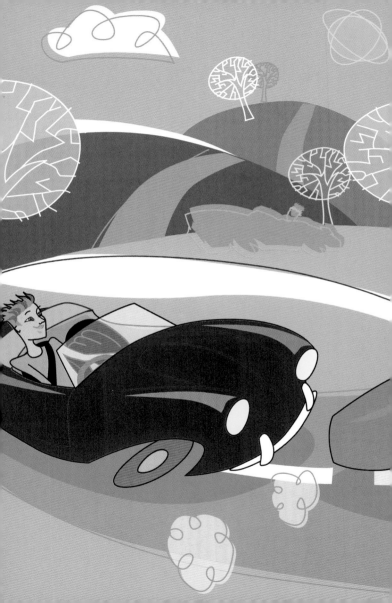

MEN RULE!

Yes, men need remedial emotional tutoring. But that doesn't mean women still can't learn a few useful lessons about life from them.

He can drive. **In general, men have a better sense of spatial relations and can judge distances better than women.** That's why they tend to do well at things like geometry, figuring out computer games and tail-gating the car in front of them. In other words, he really is more in control than he seems (sometimes, anyway).

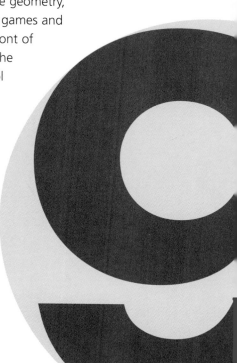

He understands what's restricted information. **Surveys have found that it's WOMEN – not men – who dish the dirt.** He'll never reveal what a great girlfriend he has because deep down he's afraid his friends might go after her (see tip 11). So men stick solely with general reports when with their friends – 'She has brown hair' – whereas women will detail everything down to the freckle on his penis.

He knows how to compete – particularly with another man over a woman. Men have a severe need to succeed and, once again, biology is to blame. **In the face of competition, a man's testosterone level soars, making him more willing to take risks.** While this overdrive can be annoying, you may not want to discourage it. According to a study conducted at Pennsylvania State University, testosterone levels of winners stay high post-battle. So if he's lucky, you may get lucky too.

The same insensitivity that makes it difficult for him to read people (go back to tip 7) keeps men in good stead for **cutting their losses when a relationship isn't working** rather than making futile attempts to work things out (hmmm – like anyone you know?).

LOSER-PROOF YOUR LIFE

Is he a relationship in the making or the breaking?
Checking out his habits is one sure way to know
you're not giving your heart to a 'going-nowhere'
kind of a guy:

Get down and boogie with him. If he lets you
set the groove, you can be sure the same will
happen in bed.

Guaranteed orgasms or guaranteed relationship?
Five signs he'd be great to Sleep/Live With:

- He never makes you hurry up/He never makes
  you wait
- He makes big delicious takes-forever-to-clean-
  up meals/He scrubs all the pans
- He lets you set the pace when you walk/When
  you start to do something – pour the coffee,
  pay for the drinks – he often says it's his turn
- Seeing him makes your pulse race/Seeing him
  puts you in a good mood
- You're on the same wavelength about condoms,
  where your hot spots are and a threesome with
  your best friend/You're on the same wavelength
  about fidelity, commitment and the future

Go shopping with him. Watch how he orders in a restaurant. If he um's and ah's between the red and blue T-shirt or always dithers over this choice of drink, he'll probably buckle under the weight of making any decision – including whether he wants a full-time girlfriend or a casual relationship.

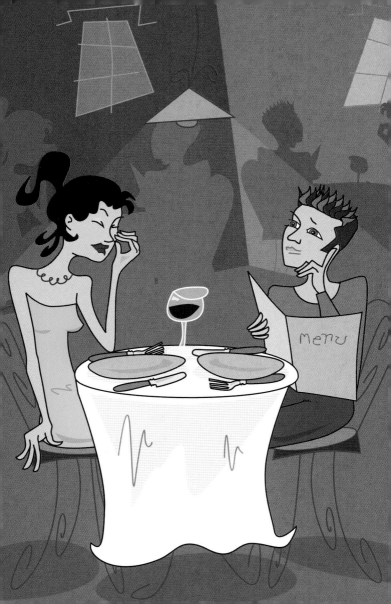

Find out how many notches he has on his bed-post.
A study in the *Journal of Personality and Social Psychology* states that **the more a guy sleeps around, the more likely his character type falls under the heading 'Creep'.**

Some adult males are men. And some are still men-in-training. Here's how to tell the difference (in other words, he should call you in about ten years):

- He knows what he wants to be doing five years down the road **VS** He's not sure what he'll be doing later tonight
- He claims to be a feminist but still insists on driving, paying for dinner and choosing the contraception **VS** He claims to be a feminist because he says you can drive (translation: he doesn't own a car with a full petrol tank), pay (translation: his credit card is maxed out) and choose the contraception (translation: it doesn't occur to him to ask about it)
- He puts you on the phone when his mother calls **VS** He pretends you're not there when his mother calls
- He starts his own business **VS** He quits his job without having another one lined up

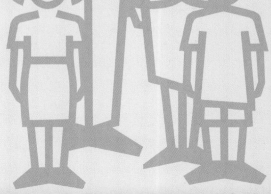

BIG FAT LIES ABOUT MEN

You can be so wrong about him.
Here's what he REALLY thinks.

OK, all you cynical, jaded, been-there, done-that,
heard-that-line, fell-for-it-anyway, how-could-I-have-
been-so-stupid, men-are-the-scum-of-the-earth
babes out there. It turns out men aren't the hound
dogs we think they are. **When a University of
Chicago survey asked men what would make
them happy, relationship, marriage and family
topped the list while sex came near the
bottom.** Maybe that's because marriage is better
for him than it is for you – men make more money,
live longer, are happier and have healthier, more and
better sex when married than women, according
to National Health and Social Life survey of
13,000 adults.

Men don't fear intimacy with women. What they fear is intimacy with the WRONG woman. **Men, in fact, seek marriage in GREATER numbers than women,** and very few remain lifelong bachelors: 94 per cent of males wed at some point in their lives – and, once a man tries marriage, he's hooked. Divorced and widowed men remarry in greater numbers.

Yes, he may be more LIKELY to cheat (see tip 56), but a Gallup Poll has uncovered a virtual epidemic of fidelity: **89 per cent of husbands report the only woman they do the wild thang with is their wife.** As heartening are the results of a Virginia Slims American Women's Opinion Poll in which more than 75 per cent of the 1,000 men surveyed thought fidelity was more important to a good marriage than a satisfying sexual relationship, financial security or having children.

You may think that men's body image issues begin and end with penis size. Wrong. The fact is, **94 per cent of men would like to change some aspect of their physical appearance.** And men who think their biceps aren't beefy enough endure the same feelings of inadequacy and depression as women who think their thighs are too thick (see tips 100 and 102 for more on what he fears body-wise).

Just because he's throwing darts three minutes after breaking up with you, don't think he isn't hurting inside. Research from the University of Michigan found that **it actually takes men about three times longer to get over a break up than women,** but it usually hits them much later. And they recover by keeping busy (see tip 113 for why). Also, although men don't cry so easily after a break-up, they do get impotent, suffer from gastrointestinal disorders, drink more, have automobile accidents and are more likely to commit suicide over a failed love affair.

22

You are more to him than his career. Asked which factors contribute most to a happy, satisfied life, nearly 2,000 men participating in the Playboy Report on American Men **ranked love second only to health.** Work came an unimpressive fifth. But the way men express their love is by providing for their family (see tip 63 to explain that one).

23

Sure, men would LIKE to have sex seven times in one day – but only once in their lives, so they can talk about it forever. Otherwise, **most are happy to call it a night after one or two body blast-offs** (and fear that YOU aren't – see tip 116).

24

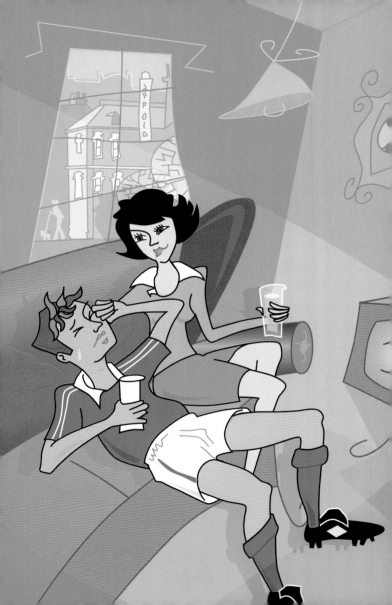

If one gender had to be labelled starry-eyed romance junkies, it would be the males. **They fall in love faster and more often than females.** Researchers have found that men are more likely than women to fall deeply in love by the fourth date, be the first to utter 'I love you' (once – see tip 51), believe that true love lasts forever and can overcome all obstacles, and are less likely to end the relationship. Awww.

Men are not breast-obsessed. Sure, they like them – a lot. But they don't need triple-letter sizes. When young men were asked to rate front-view line drawings of female physiques for attractiveness in an Archives of Sexual Behavior study, ratings were unaffected by breast size.

Men get soppy. But not over *The English Patient*. Sit with him **when his favourite team loses, however, and you'll see him weep furiously.**

PSYCH HIM OUT

Sneaky tactics guaranteed to make him want what you want – to stay with you.

28 Always be ready to leave. **Men thrive on competition** (reread tip 11) and knowing you aren't totally committed cranks him up a gear into making you want him.

29 If you're looking for a long-term relationship, keep your party dress on until he dials again. Studies show that while the average man will have sex on a first date in a heartbeat, **he doesn't want to get involved with a woman willing to sleep with him on the first date** because he thinks she's doing this with other men (leading to tip 57).

30 **Bake him a pumpkin pie.** Apparently this scent (along with lavender, black liquorice and doughnuts) spikes penile blood flow, according to a Chicago's Smell & Taste Treatment and Research Foundation study.

Get ahead. According to a University of Utah study, men are 50 per cent more likely to respond to a personal ad where the woman describes herself as ambitious rather than attractive or slim.

Go on The Pill (once you know he's safe). The reality is that he doesn't care about using condoms because he isn't as afraid of AIDS, STDs and pregnancy as you are. And research backs him up. **Women are TWO TIMES more likely to be infected through sex with a man who's infected than a man would be through sleeping with a woman who's infected.**

Say you'd rather stay at home tonight. Researchers at the University of Illinois found that **men are basically nesters,** happiest at home, even while doing the chores. (Women are more likely to go into a joy trance away from la casa.) The reason? He feels more in control in his own surroundings, giving him home court advantage.

Stop dieting. According to University of Texas study, **men love your curves.**

Make it thigh-high and lacy. According to one survey, **lingerie ranked way over toys, games and sharing fantasies as the average male's favourite erotic aid** (by the way, the wowza-wowza combo is high heels and lots of make-up).

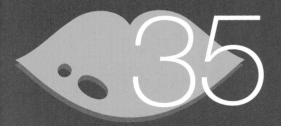
35

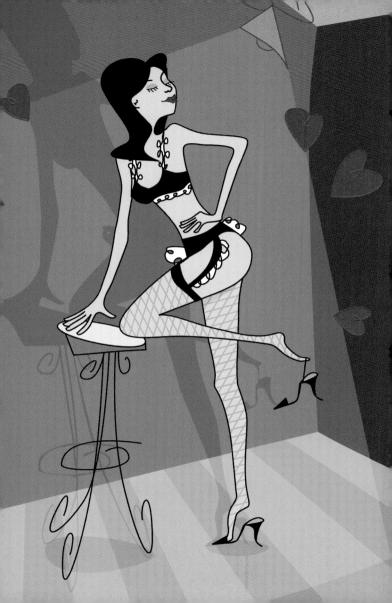

his **heart**

As a gender, men have a lot to answer for. Not just warfare, topless models and Arnold Schwarzenegger, but all their pitiable excuses, the total selfishness, the strategic hot-and-cold attitude – all quiet little ways of treating a relationship as anything other than the delicate little soufflé it is.

However, splicing jokes aside, it's clear that the one thing **ALL** men want is a relationship (or at least say they do when you get them alone after a few beers and a particularly bad day). They just don't want to initiate it, work at it, talk about it or think about it. The reality is, men are not trying to avoid **ALL** women – they're trying to avoid all but one. The One.

To understand what makes a man see a woman as the one he wants to marry and other insights into his true desires, read on.

MAN WATCHING

How well do you pick up the silent signals
a man sends?

When a guy says he'll call you, it's hard to tell
if he means it (see tip 59 for more on this), but
**something in the way he moves can provide
a few clues:**

- He looks at you: Your bust, that is. And
  then he makes contact with your eyes
- He ignores you: No guy actively avoids female
  attention, unless he's already enjoyed yours and
  decided not to go there again. So this is his
  pathetic way of trying to make you think he's
  cool as opposed to desperate
- He stands so close to you that you know what
  he had for breakfast: He's trying to tell you
  that he's attracted to you, but in a way that
  suggests he may be telling you what to wear
  and who you can hang out with in the future
- He thrusts his chest at you: This is an instinctive
  move all males make to attract a mate – in
  short, he wants you

Turn the page for more …

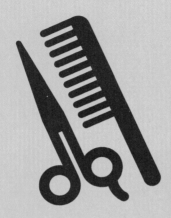

- He grooms himself, patting
  his hair, adjusting his clothes,
  tugging his chin: He's saying
  'Look at me! Look at me!
  Look at me!'
- He's rubbing his own arm
  or chest: He's thinking,
  'Me, Tarzan; You, Jane'
- He touches your arm: He feels
  touchy-feely towards you – get
  ready for a kiss
- He's sitting with legs wide open:
  He's an alpha-male, splaying
  what he's got and saying,
  'Come and get it!'

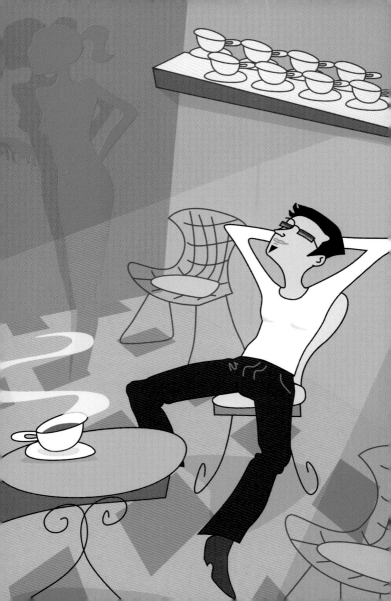

You're clearly giving him the Yes signal but he still doesn't make a move (dammit!). The reason is that he doesn't have a clue. **The way you run your fingers through your hair might mean you want him to kiss you like you've never been kissed before or it might mean your scalp is itchy. Who knows?** He certainly doesn't (see tip 7). So, not to put too fine a point on it, if you want him, take him. He won't mind.

37

38

It turns out that the Crotch Grab isn't just his way of saying, 'Check me out, I'm da man!' **Testicle adjustment is sometimes necessary for the sake of comfort.** These boys get bounced around a lot during the day and need to be put back in place.

ACCESSORIZE!

Girls, it's a jungle out there. He may be tall, cuter than Brad Pitt, hold a job, have ready cash and practically smell of sex, but STILL be a commitment-phobic two-timing jerk. Pay attention to his trimmings – according to psychologists, **things like his favourite colour and snack are what give away his inner bloke.**

HE SMELLS OF …
- **Citrus:** Likes hanging with the lads
- **Spice:** Adventure seeker who may suddenly disappear from your life without warning
- **English Leather:** Dependable – he'll always call when he says he will
- **Floral:** He wants to overpower you
- **Musk:** A sensualist. Count on lots of foreplay.
- **No scent:** Macho man. Comes in two types: 1) manly sexist; and 2) grungy slob. You'll smell the difference

POSITION YOURSELF IN …
- **Missionary:** A traditionalist
- **Doggy:** He likes submissive women
- **You on top:** He likes a woman who takes control
- **You sitting on his lap:** He stays active while you stay in charge (we'll take him!)

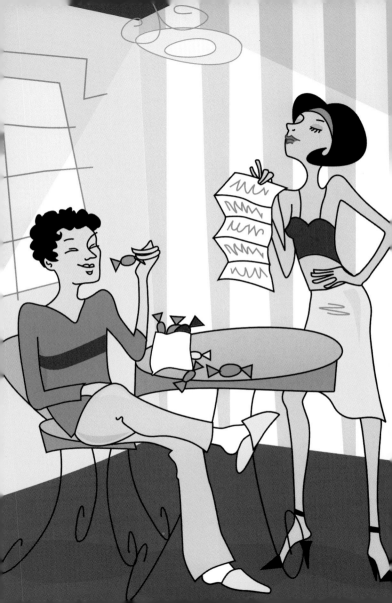

HE DRESSES …
- **Bottom Up** (knickers, socks, trousers, shoes, shirt, tie): Well-grounded – he'll always pay the rent and keep his promises
- **Top Down** (shirt, tie, knickers, trousers, socks, shoes): Hates details. Frequently misplaces keys and forgets to call you. But he'll blow his rent money on sexy lingerie for you
- **Varies:** Changeable – might not be dependable

HIS SNACK ATTACKS …
- **Crisps:** A social butterfly. Enjoy the ride but You'll need patience (and tips 28–35) to net him
- **Candy:** Still a kid at heart. Sounds like fun … until you have to pay all the bills yet again because he's spent his salary on boy toys
- **Sandwiches:** Tough and determined, he'll work hard to please you
- **Chocolate:** Since choccie contains chemicals that bring on a natural high, his craving for it could signal a need for instant gratification – which won't satisfy your need for commitment

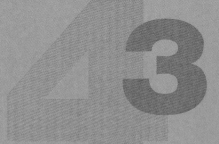

HIS OUTER BEAST …

- **German Shepherd-type Dog:** A crotch sniffer
- **Labrador-type Dog:** Friendly and fun, but needs lots of exercise
- **Corgi-type Dog:** Annoyingly smart but good at respecting space
- **Rottweiler-type Dog:** Protective jealous type – potential abuser
- **Persian Cat:** Hard to please and a bit lazy
- **Short-Haired Cat:** Self-confident
- **Bird/Fish/Any Reptile:** Will back off as soon as it seems you're getting close
- **Rodent:** A secret trainspotter
- **Menagerie:** Easy-going, nurturing and social, but also has lots of demands on his attention

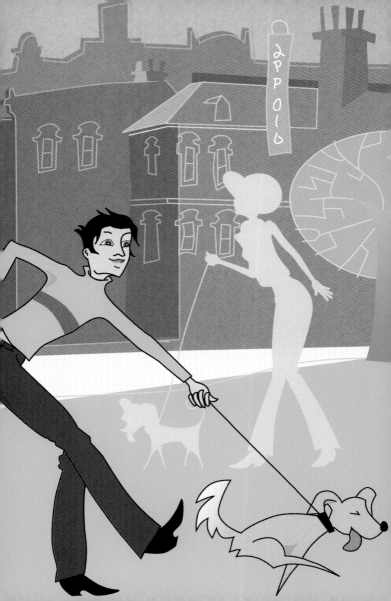

Read the sports page for a handle on his nookie stamina. **New studies show that an avid sport fan's testosterone level shoots up 2 per cent after a victory,** leaving him ready for a particularly passionate lovemaking session.Of course, if the team loses, you can always console him with some replay-worthy sex.

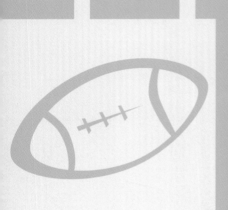

Check out his nails. If they're creamy and transparent, he's likely to be a perspirer because the excess moisture changes the nail – which could also mean a nervous personality.

HIS PET GIRLFRIEND PEEVES

Do these and he'll behave like a cornered rat – bolting at the first opportunity.

Talk dirty – about an ex. When you're in love, the desire to open the book to your life is intoxicating. Just remember: men are often insecure sexually (skip on to tip 108) and hearing you've done it all with some other guy can be unsettling. A man's checklist of need-to-know information is short: 'Do you have an STD? Are you on trial for a violent crime? Are you married?' Beyond that, he just doesn't wanna know.

Share too much: He doesn't want you to dish all to your friends, no matter how adorable it was that he cried when his team won the championship. (On the other hand, any tales of his amazing stud abilities are fine for general broadcast.)

Push his head down during sex. He'll get there when he gets there. And he **WILL** get there. Recent polls reveal that muff diving is a top guy activity (right after boning).

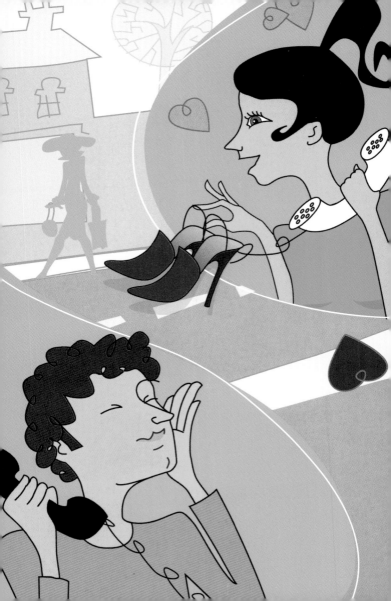

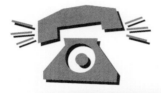

Put him through endless chat on the phone. **There's only one type of conversation he gets into – it's called phone sex.**

49

Constantly ask if he loves you. If he's told you once, then that sticks until he makes an exit (see tip 65).

5 ♥ **5**

Discuss the future. You're together – isn't that enough? Do you have to talk about it all the time? (If you let the 'F' word slip, don't worry – go back to tip 28) .

WHY MEN STAY

What makes a man get down on bended knee.

You're like the girl next door. **Men divide women into two categories – those you screw and those you marry.** He likes wild and crazy – but not to spend the rest of his life with. According to studies, when men are just on the trawl, they seek the Pamela Anderson formula of sexiness. But when they're looking for someone to marry, it's more likely to be someone who is beautiful in their own mind.

52 53

You caught him at the right 'Tom' moment. There are Toms (as in Cruise) and there are Toms (as in Hanks). One is forever a boy; the other, though boyish, is definitely a man – a man who realizes he wants to marry, have children and settle down. (See tip 17 to decide which yours is).

54

Keep him guessing. **The number one male fantasy is sex with lots of women.** So when you constantly surprise him, he never has a chance to get bored. However, since there are only so many sexual positions, scents, camisoles, lipsticks, breath-freshener tricks and so on in the universe, spread them out over a chunk of time to keep him interested.

55

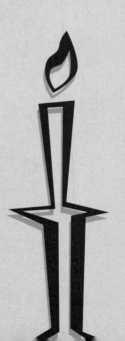

Making love. Researchers at Bowling Green University found that men rate this one of their top romantic acts, along with giving flowers, kissing, taking a walk and candlelight dinners. The one thing they hardly mentioned? Saying/hearing the phrase, 'I love you'.

HIS CHEATING HEART

What makes a guy roam outside his home turf.

A worldwide study of over 37 different cultures established what you knew all along – **men cheat more than women.** The dilemma: they also want to marry a woman with little sexual experience. The reason: they have a biological imperative to spread their own genes but don't want to end up supporting some other bloke's little genes.

You suspect yours is not the only station he is servicing. According to research on an average cheat's profile, here's how to know for sure:

- He refuses to consider living together, even though you spend all your time together
- He swept you off your feet (he's a serial romantic)
- He's over-detailed when explaining where he's been/who with and for how long (he's getting his story straight)
- He consistently heads straight for the bathroom before you've even kissed him hello (he's removing evidence)
- He develops an incredible new sexual technique (this one might make it almost worth it)

According to a University of Indiana study, **men are more likely to stray more when:**

- There's a baby in the house (not him)
- Someone else gets ahead of him career-wise (he thinks, 'I'm a loser')
- YOU get ahead of him career-wise (he thinks, 'I'm a wussy loser')
- He has a big win (he thinks he's so cool that everyone loves him and wants him)
- He starts losing his hair – or anything else that reminds him he's getting older, fatter, uglier
- He falls in love (it's his cute way of saying he really cares about you – so much that it scares him right into another woman's arms)
- A woman makes it clear she wants him
- He suspects you're cheating

58

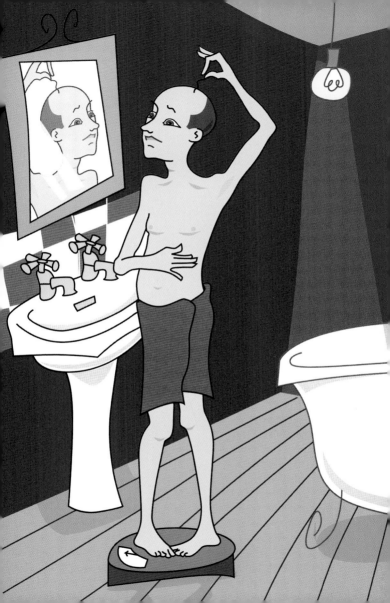

his **tongue**

There's an old joke about a wife who nags her husband, 'Tell me how you feel'. Finally, the husband blurts, 'I feel … I feel … like watching television'.

The awful truth is, most men have no idea how they feel at any given time. Studies show that men use language to establish difference, separateness and independence (exactly the opposite of women, who talk to connect). So demanding that he talk to you is guaranteed to make him squirm and start rambling about whether new Cheerios really are improved.

Here are the answers and explanations to his biggest verbal 'Huhs?' (you'll be speaking like a native in no time).

MAN-SPEAK

An at-a-glance guide to his love talk.

A slew of research has established that men and women use language in different ways. For women, talk is the glue that holds relationships together. To men, conversation is a means, not an end. They don't even like talking to each other that much – two guys can watch a game in silence for four hours and walk away feeling they've bonded. **When men do use words, it's primarily doublespeak to stay on top.** Here's how to make sense of the favourite phrases he uses for different stages of your union:

WHEN YOU'RE DATING

He says: So maybe we could get together or something?
He means: I think you're really hot and want to ask you out, but I'm too chicken to say so

He says: Nothing about seeing you again
He means: His mojo wasn't rising

He says: You're a really good person
He means: You'll never see him again

He says: Let's be friends
He means: You're not my type, but could you set me up with your hot friend?

He says: I'll call you
He means: I really mean to call but I'm scared you'll say Yes, we'll go out and it will be a letdown. Or worse, what if it's not? Do I want to go through all the hassle of dating? Get married? Have kids? Aaahhhh!

He says: We're dating
He means: We've spent at least five nights together, at least one of which has ended in sexual contact. But in no way are we exclusive

He says: We're seeing each other
He means: It's down to you and one other woman

He says: I think we should date exclusively
He means: I'm scared that if I don't make things more permanent, you'll date someone else

WHEN HE WANTS SEX

He says: This is our third date, isn't it?
He says: Is it warm out or just me?
He says: What time do you go to work in the morning?
He says: You think it's true what they say about oysters?
He means: I WANT SEX

He says (in the middle of a great orgasm): I love you
He means: I love that incredible thing you are doing with your finger/tongue/body right now

He says (immediately after making love): It'll be great to show you the house I grew up in (or anything else that smacks of the future)
He means: Are you thinking about your ex and how much better he was than me?

He says: We haven't spoken for ages and I've been thinking about you
He means: I haven't gotten laid in almost three months

He says: I'm not looking to get serious
He means: I just want a little nookie

He says: How many guys have you been with?
He means: I'm the best, right?

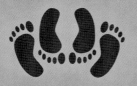

WHEN YOU'RE A COUPLE

He says: I really like you
He means: I think I am falling in love but if I say that word, there is no going back

He says (in middle of a date): It'll be great to show you the house I grew up in (or anything else that smacks of the future)
He means: See above

He says: 'Girlfriend' and he's not doing a Ru Paul imitation
He means: You've made him breakfast, he fixed your car and his buddies aren't allowed to come on to you

He says: Nothing's wrong. I'm fine
He means: God, I know you want to talk about my day and all my interrelationships with my colleagues and boss and the guy who drives my bus, but I am home now and I just want to drink ten beers, eat a bag of chips for dinner and zone out

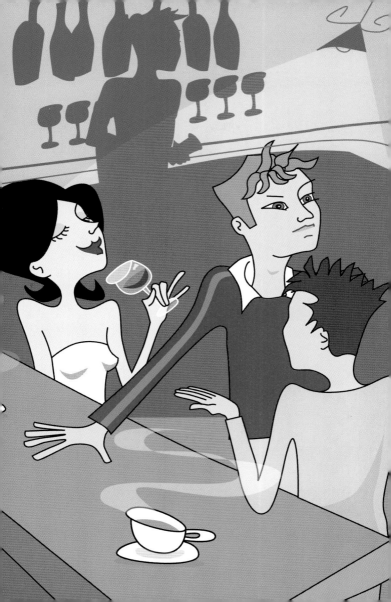

He says: Maybe we need to slow down
He means: Maybe you need to slow down

He says: I don't know what I want
He means: I don't want you

He says: I need some space
He means: I'm about this close to dumping
you but I haven't worked up the nerve yet

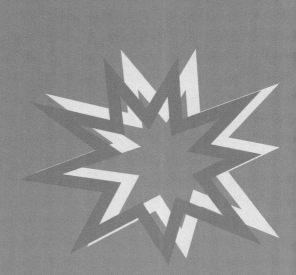

He says: You're an amazing woman
He means: You're an amazing woman

He says: I love you
He means: You make me incredible happy
whenever we are together. I think you may be
The One

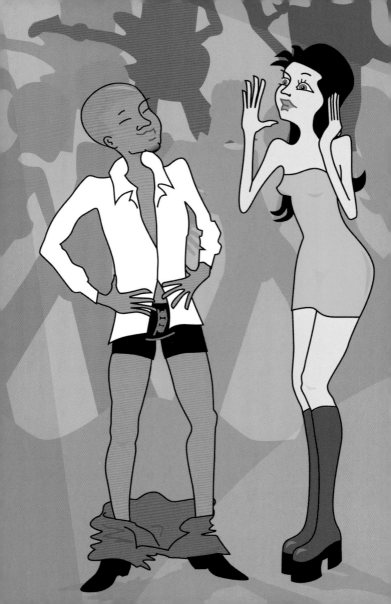

As noted in the first tip, **men don't always hear everything you're saying.** Which means he's not always getting your message:

You say (after being introduced): Do you know this band?
He hears: I want you now

You say: What do you do?
He hears: Are you making enough money to make you marriage material?

You say: My ex is a crazy stalker who won't stop calling me. He scares me
He hears: I'm still in love with my ex

You say: What are we doing Saturday night?
He hears: I want all your time for the rest of your life

You say (after making love): That was really nice
He hears: That was the best sex of my life. Let's do it again!

TOP LIES MEN TELL WOMEN

- But I TRIED to call
- I didn't get the message
- I didn't notice what she looked like
- Sex isn't the most important thing
- I'll be careful
- We'll talk about it later
- I'm not mad
- I could fall in love with you in a minute (wait a minute and ask him how he feels now)

TALKING HIS TALK

How to talk to a man so he understands you.

Men can only take directions one at a time.
So if you want him to go into the kitchen and get
you a cup of tea, make it a two-part request (this
also applies to when you are in bed with him).

62

**When men bother to use words, it's to inspire
action** (whereas women communicate to bond). So
if a guy insults another guy, he automatically thinks
he wants to fight. And if you say you like his shirt, he
thinks, 'Cool – she wants to jump my bones!'

63

University of Houston psychologists investigating
why **men keep things bottled up** found it was to
maintain power in a relationship – when they don't
talk, their partner is left guessing. You do the same
and he'll be putty in your hands (see tip 54 for why).

64

**Men don't want to talk about the relationship.
They just want to do it** (in his mind, if he didn't
love you, he'd leave). Here's how he thinks: 'If we
need to talk about the relationship, it must be broken.
If it's broken, it means it's doomed. I'm outta here.'

65

A man will say, 'I'm fine', even when being tortured by Zulu warriors. **It's in his nature not to reveal weakness because that betrays vulnerability, which comes off as lack of status,** according to research by evolutionary psychologist David Buss. In short, he's worried you'll think he's a weed if he can't solve his problems without his Superwoman girlfriend coming to his aid.

There are certain words his tongue seem to trip over – like 'girlfriend', 'love' and 'commitment'. But since men are action-driven (see tip 65), **it's really more important what he does than what he says.** You know your man really loves you if he:

- Lets you drive his car (especially his new SUV)
- Assumes you're spending the weekend together
- Introduces you to his friends
- Stops wearing his 'If you're not wasted, the day is' T-shirt, because he knows you hate it
- Calls for absolutely no reason
- Wants to talk after sex

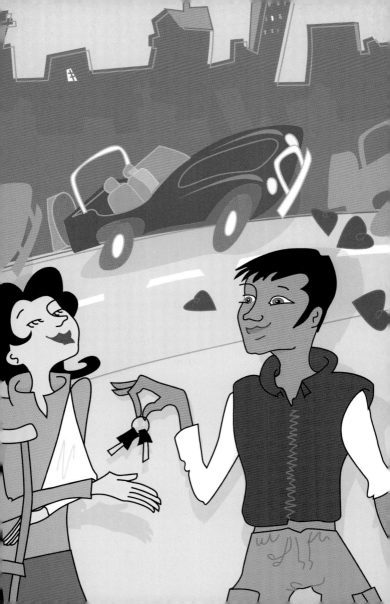

Here's what he really doesn't want to ever hear from you (and probably won't hear anyway – see tip 1):

- Honey, we have to talk: No, YOU have to talk – and talk and talk and talk

- What are you thinking about?: His feelings, like his answers, will be simple. So if you are lying in post-coital comfort and he answers, 'Pizza', he really means he is thinking about pizza and not that you have skin that resembles pizza or you look like you've eaten one too many pies in your life

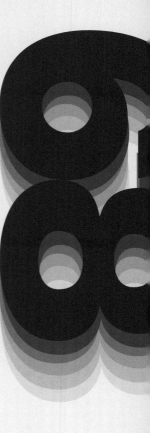

- Do you think that girl is pretty?: He thinks that if he even hesitates to say no, it will kill his chances of sex that night – or any other night
- I want to get married: He already assumes this is what you want, he just doesn't want to hear it. So you only have to notify him if this is NOT the case
- How do I look – honestly?: Honestly, you look wonderful to him. That's why he's with you

his **private parts**

What's his world view? Depends. Is he: About to have an orgasm? In the midst of having one? Just finished having one?

If it sometimes seems that a man thinks with his penis, it's because he does. Hormones dictate that he has one biological function: to deposit sperm. In anyone, any time, anywhere. In short, the essential distinction between a man and a woman can be summed up in a single word: testosterone.

Now that you understand his primary driving force, it's time to get a handle on that holiest of appliances: his genitals. To be honest, most women don't have a clue as to what's going on down there. You know men pee, zip, tuck, scratch and, every once in a lucky while (they think), they spelunk – and sometimes it seems all at once. But don't worry. There's nothing to programme, no wires to splice. Not a shred of assembly is required.

So roll up your sleeves, and turn down the sheets.

BELOW THE BELT

A do-it-yourselfer's guide to the worldwide family of penis owners.

A man with a big nose just has a big nose. **Actually, the size of his tool depends on his background rather than the size of any other part of his anatomy.** Here's the score, according to a study published by the Charles Darwin Research Institute:

- **Black men:** 16 to 20 cm (6¼ to 7⅞ in) long and 5 cm (2 in) diameter when erect
- **White men:** 14 to 15 cm (5½ to 5⅞ in) long and 3.3 to 4 cm (1⅜ to 1⅝ in) diameter when erect
- **Asian men:** 10 to 14 cm (4 to 5½ in) long and 3.2 cm (1¼ in) diameter when erect

Get out your stopwatch. Kinsey studies found that **it generally takes a twentysomething three to five minutes to stand to attention** (warning: this reaction time at least doubles with age).

Cool your heels (and other body parts). After orgasm, a man enters a refractory or down period where he has to wait anywhere from five minutes (in his teens) to a day (if he's 50+) until the next stiffy comes along.

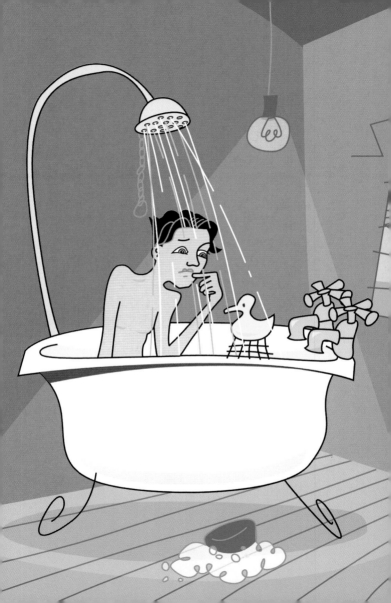

Read washing
instructions. The
following can shrink
a relaxed penis by
5 cm (2 in) or more:
cold weather, chilly
baths or showers,
sexual activity, illness,
exhaustion, excitement
(nonsexual). Seems it's
a protective mechanism.
**His penis needs a nice
warm environment
or else it instinctively
goes into hiding.**

73

Three things even he doesn't know about his sperm:

- His sperm has legs. It can live for 5 to 7 days inside you
- It would take a sperm 30 minutes to travel across this page
- A teaspoon of ejaculate can contain more than 600 million sperm (although this is enough to populate the UK ten times over, there's only a 15 per cent chance that one of them will score a direct hit). The average amount of semen per ejaculation increases if he downs a few beers, hasn't had sex since Sylvester Stallone had a hit movie and eats zinc and vitamin C

He may not feel your pain, but he feels another guy's. **The one sure place a man hurts is his groin.** The area is so chockablock full of ultrasensitive nerve endings that they even respond when someone gets a poke in the privates.

74

He gets blue when he doesn't have sex. When a man is aroused, **blood floods not only to the penis but to the entire area.** The longer he stays aroused, the longer the blood stays there. Newer blood is red, but older blood, which has less oxygen, is blue, giving his balls a bluish hue. However, it's not harmful, so don't let him use this as a seduction line.

Men as embryos were also women. After testosterone is added, they become boys – but with a few souvenirs left over from his drag queen stint. Such as nipples, a hymen (sitting uselessly near the prostate gland) and a vagina (called vagina masculina, it's a paltry piece of tissue dangling from his bladder). This is all offset by a keen interest in motor sports.

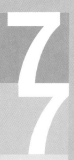

HIS BEST FRIEND

His penis made him do it
(so don't take it personally).

A recent Kaiser study
found that **59 per cent
of single men didn't
use a condom the last
time they had sex.** The
top reason: no quickies on
the steps (that is, a lack of
spontaneity); complaints
that wearing a rubber was
like eating a steak covered
in clingfilm (saranwrap)
followed a close second.

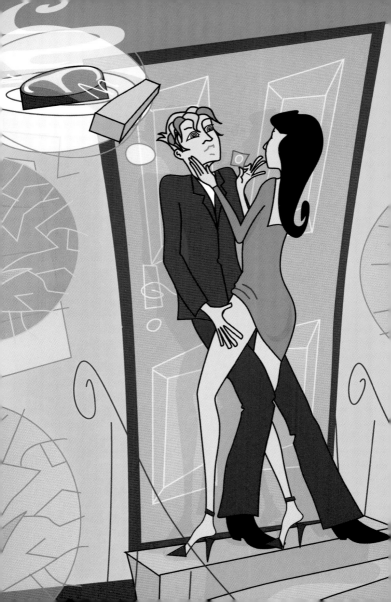

If he's a gawker, he may just be following his basic instincts. **Men are programmed to respond to visual stimuli like porn, erotic undies and gorgeous babes in order to spread sperm and propagate the species.** Which is why the quickest way to a man's groin is through his eyes (see tip 87 for how to make him look).

The male member has over 200 different 'official' pet names; the most popular being Mr Happy (he wishes!). Though medical science is still sceptical, men name their penises because they believe the penis has a brain completely separate from their own. How else can they explain why they choose to follow its suggestions on major life choices?

He often has sex with the one he loves. Sex therapists joke that **90 per cent of men masturbate at least once a week and the other 10 per cent are lying about it.** Call it McSex – jerking off is quick, convenient and satisfying without G-spot worries.

DON'T TOUCH

What makes a makes a guy lose his lust.

Common sense tells us that a man may not be erect because he's not excited. But impotence – otherwise known in slang as erectile dysfunction – is often separate from lack of sexual desire. **In fact, in the under-forties set, it is almost always the result of TOO MUCH desire,** which leads to a fear of failure and then to failure itself. (But you knew that already, didn't you?)

No work, no wood. To test the effects of stress on sexual function, researchers had a group of jobless men and a group of employed men watch adult movies. Stress was induced by telling the guys they'd have to talk about their own sexual behaviour and fantasies afterwards to a group of students. When they knew that later they'd have to spill their guts sexually, **the jobless men had poorer erections during the videos than the employed men**. Conclusion: There must be a better way for the unemployed to see free porn.

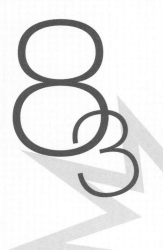

University of Houston studies have found that anger makes his desire wane while anxiety (they used the threat of electric shock!) **actually increases the size of his erections** (stress could make it go either way). Conclusion: Forget about good make-up sex, get him nervous with tip 28 and stop worrying about stressing him out.

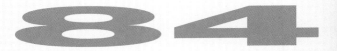

Depression is the most common clinical dampener of lust. Even mild levels of the blues can make his noodle droop.

SEXUAL CRAVINGS

No, lots of instant sex with boatloads of women does **NOT** top the list.

The turn-on of a woman who gets the sexual ball rolling can hardly be under-estimated (with special bonus points going to those who've tried the greet-him-telling-him-you're-not-wearing-underwear game). Putting his hand somewhere that would get you arrested if you did it in the supermarket goes a long way towards appeasing his secret terror that no matter how deeply attracted he is to you, you won't like him (see tip 103).

Because **the penis is where men feel pleasure most intensely,** you can never pay too much attention to it – love it, adore it, worship it. See tips 89–93 for some strategy notes.

Because men are much more visual creatures than women (see tip 78), **he doesn't just want to look during sex – he needs to.** If you really want to make his tongue hang out, do it with the lights on.

85
88
86
87

Similarly, let him see himself naked. Researchers had men sit naked in a chair with and without a board covering their laps. They then watched some porno.

Watching the steamy films, they had the firmest erections when not wearing the board. The point of all this: **Men become more stimulated if they can actually see that they are stimulated.** But don't try this when you are at the cinema.

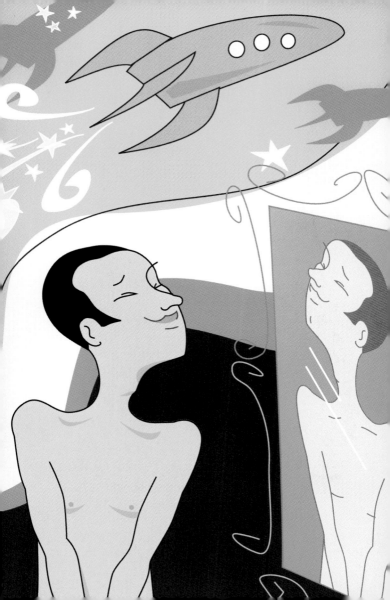

HOW TO TOUCH A NAKED MAN
Flip his switch and turn him on.

89

Your man has his own G-spot. Owing to its location at the base of the penis, a man's erection is more-or-less anchored upon the prostate, a randy nerve-rich gland so sensitive it even secretes fluid during arousal and ejaculation.

Best Move: Slip a well-lubricated finger through the rectum and probe the rounded back wall of the prostrate. When you feel a firm, round, walnut-size lump, gently caress it while stroking his penis.

A man's erection doesn't end at the base of the penis. There's a railroad junction full of nerves in the perineum, that smooth triangle of flesh between the base of his penis and his anus which, when pressed, will send him straight into an orgasmic swoon.

Best Move: Gently rub the spot with the pad of your finger or thumb. (Pressing really hard with one forceful push can actually stop him from peaking, so be careful.)

90

Stroking his frenulum – the vertical ridge that extends from the tip to the shaft of the penis – will hit his moan zone. Not only are there more nerve endings there, but the skin is also extremely thin.
Best Move: Clenching your pelvic muscles just as he pulls out will give his F-Spot a massage.

Many men are surprised to discover the range and depth of the sensation when you stroke their raphe, the visible line along the centre of the scrotum. They may even end up ejaculating sooner than they (and you) planned.
Best Move: Excite this lust locale by gently running your fingertips along it.

Don't forget his ego – a little stroking goes a long way towards making him relaxed and open to intimacy.
Best Move: Make him feel that you want him (see tip 117).

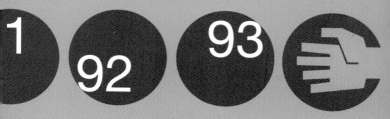

1 92 93

CAN A MAN EVER HAVE BAD SEX?

Five facts about his Big O – this stuff is so secret even he doesn't know it!

Timing is everything. In short, when he's about to come, let him go with the flow (unless he's aiming for tip 96). If he blows those final few seconds before ejaculation, his orgasm will be a dud, leading to tip 97.

It may seem as though he can have an orgasm just rubbing against a tree. But it's not that simple. **A satisfying experience for a man involves lots of pressure.** That's why the hard thrusting at the end of intercourse is so important. It's what shoves him over the edge (see tips 91 and 92 for how to handle his penis).

He can also have more than one orgasm. In a State University of New York Health Science Center study, men aged 22 to 56 had from three to ten orgasms during extended bouts of sexual stimulation without ejaculation. Their favourite moment: Stopping stimulation just at the brink of orgasm, then starting again once they regained control.

In men, orgasm and ejaculation are not the same thing. The first is the physical and mental release of sexual tension while the second refers to the release of semen, which can sometimes occur without orgasm. In other words, he can fake it too (and 43 per cent have done so at least once).

97

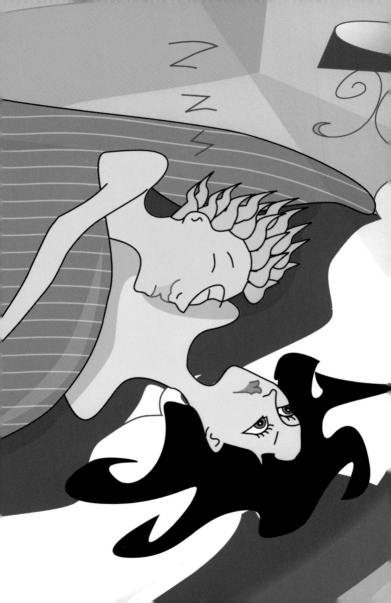

The real reason men snooze after sex: It seems that oxytocin, a hormone that stimulates women's orgasmic contractions and his erection and ejaculation, also causes drowsiness. But because women's bodies normally contain more of it, they may be less sensitive to its surges. Men, on the other hand, fall into a drunken stupor from it.

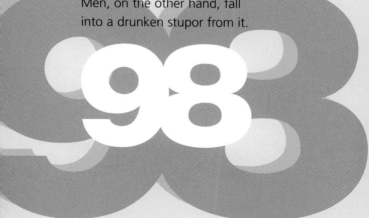

98

his **hair**

Although men may lead you to believe they can handle absolutely anything, the reality is that your average guy has lots of fears. Even the biggest, strongest he-man can turn into a trembling powder-puff of anxiety given the right circumstances.

And nowhere – nowhere – is a man more likely to have a meltdown than in how he relates to you. Men panic when something threatens their sense of self, and most men's self-concept (as you probably guessed) is rooted in their sex life (read: penis). Put another way, guys freak out over anything and everything from asking you out to making whoopee with you.

Here are the top fears that plague men (not that they'll ever tell you). Use your knowledge wisely.

LIFE CONCERNS

Bottom line: Being a man is a scary business.

He's scared of violating the Code of Guys: A man will not appear to be ruled by **his girlfriend, his mother, his boss** or anything other than his penis for fear of being ousted from the group.

He's worried about his thread count: **Most men would rather be castrated than go bald.** The trouble is that everyone can see his hair all the time, while penises manifest themselves only to a chosen few. No one ever had a thinning penis.

He's afraid of you: This can be traced back millions of years to men being awed by things women can do that they can't – menstruate, have children, do more than two things at the same time (if you think men have made any progress after 2.5 million years, try saying tampon in a roomful of guys).

He has height-challenged fears. **More than one in three men report that they'd like to be taller.**

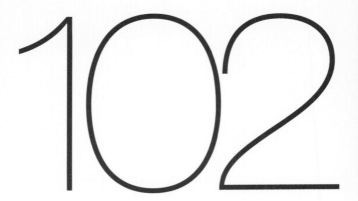

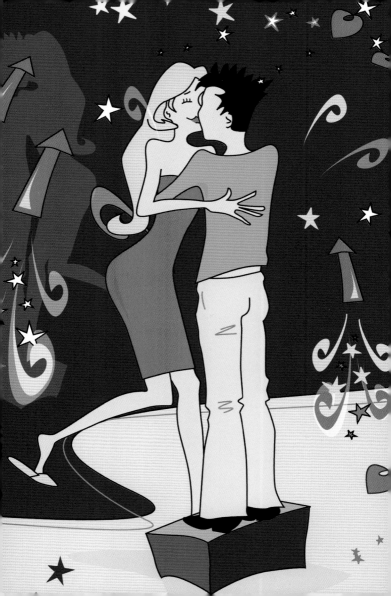

LOVE WORRIES

The more he is into you, the more scared he gets.

His biggest dating doubts:

- **Making the first move:** Because men are often expected to make the first move, we assume they're used to being turned down. Not so. Whether he's 14 or 34, calling you for a date is like phoning the undertaker to arrange his own funeral (see tip 59). Surveys have found that men feel they're putting their manhood on the line every time they ask you out (a little appreciation on your part goes a long way for him)

- **What to talk about:** In his mind, silence equals death. Whenever there's a pause in the conversation he thinks, 'It's over! She's noticed my receding hairline (see tip 100)'

- **Whether to smooch:** Go back to Making The First Move, above

- **Calling you for a second date:** Making a woman wait for the follow-up call is a man's way of gaining back the upper hand. Unfortunately this leaves you in the position of not knowing whether the phone is silent because he doesn't like you, or because he does (see tip 59 for help on whether to call)

He's scared of settling because:
Part One: What if Pamela Anderson calls? No matter how incredible you are (plenty), he's haunted by the possibility of tip 114.
Part Two: He may like you TOO much. Ergo – he wants nothing more to do with you. This is because he either fears a) you won't like him as much; or b) you will, shortly followed by quitting your job, having 16 children, five dogs, demanding a six-bedroom mansion and so on – all of which means he will work for the rest of his life in order to support you.
Part Three: Getting into a committed relationship will tame him. And it will. A Syracuse University study found that testosterone levels are high in single men, decrease in married men and rise in divorced men. This is possibly because single men need to be more aggressive to be able to compete for women, while married men can mellow out because they have the goods and can therefore get on with tip 3.
Part Four: You'll find out that he really does want marriage (although maybe not to you). Go back to tip 18.
Part Five: He will have to start putting the toilet seat down.

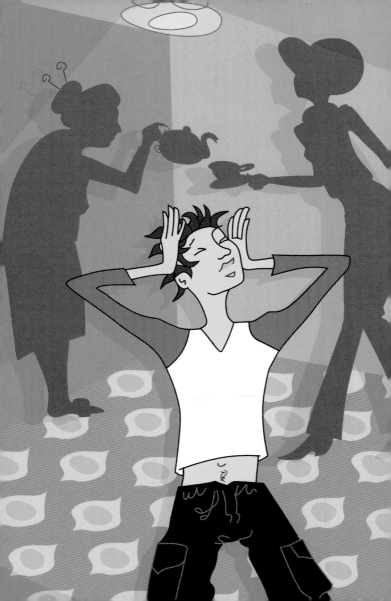

He's worried you'll **cheat on him**. Seems it's men who have the real raging hormones. A New Zealand study found that because of his high testosterone levels, he's still prone to jealousy freak-outs and suspicion. So next time he pulls his third degree act, just tell yourself it must be his time of the month.

He's anxious you'll **break up with him**. (see tip 22).

He's terrified **his mother will like you**. Or not like you. Sorry – you can't win this one.

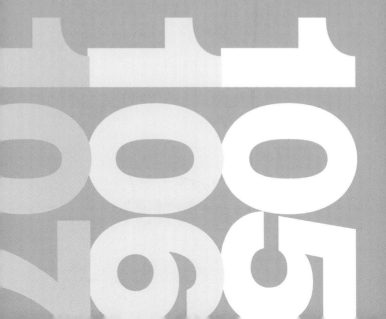

MEET MR SOFTEE
What pushes his sexual panic buttons.

Bulletin: **Self-esteem ain't just a girl thing.** Crippling as an unreturned phone call … able to fell tall erections with a single 'It's OK, let's just go to sleep' … devastating as the seventeenth mention of the solicitor-rock-climber-gourmet chef at your gym … in truth, it's amazing he's ever able to perform at all. Bringing us to …

He has opening-night jitters. Is it big enough? Will it stay up long enough? **The reality is that men are so often preoccupied with how they'll appear and perform as sexual partners that they're rarely scrutinizing women as much as women fear they're being scrutinized** (in one poll of over 3,000 men, anxiety as to whether he has what it takes to please a woman was the top fear). The possibility that a female he fancies may not want to kiss him, sleep with him, sleep with him a second time or eventually fall in love with him is often enough to make men bail emotionally (explaining why he's uncomfortable and silent the minute after he sleeps with you, even though he is clearly nuts about you – see tip 67 for other ways to tell he's falling hard).

Condoms (see tip 77).

Coming too quickly (causing him to revert to tip 109).

Impotence (see tip 81)

He's worried you'll figure out he doesn't know the way. Men don't ask for directions in bed for the same reason they don't ask for directions in general. Hormones. According to research by evolutionary psychologist Helen Fisher, PhD, communication is linked to the hormone oestrogen. Since men have significantly less oestrogen, they're less verbal and more action-oriented. **That means it's up to you to give your honey a helping hand when it comes to locating your hot spots.**

He thinks he'll never get any again after age 30. According to the University of Chicago's General Social Survey, men have the most sexual intercourse between the ages of 18 and 29. The majority of men in this age-group report bumping bones one or two times a week. After that, the slow, inexorable slide begins. So by age 70, you can expect to be getting lucky only once a month.

He's afraid you'll want to cuddle after sex. Let's face it, **for men, intercourse culminating with orgasm is the main goal.** Everything else is like little paper umbrellas in drinks – fussy and getting in the way of (in this case, his need for – see tip 98) sleep.

115

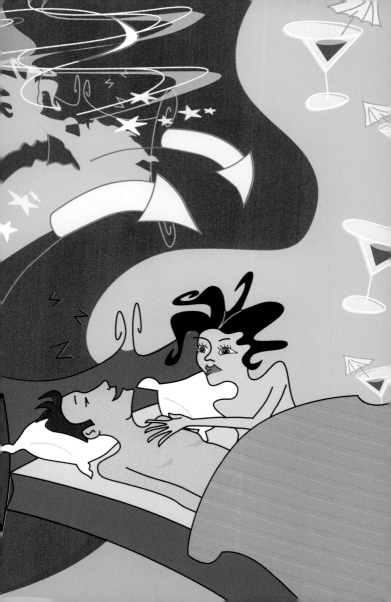

116 Two words – marathon sex. Guys know women dig tons of foreplay. The problem is, **they confuse body caresses with actual penetration and think you want intercourse to last longer than the re-release of *Apocalypse Now*.** And if they don't go the distance, they fear they'll be labelled a lame lover and you'll therefore seek out a man blessed with more stamina. Result: Every encounter has him straining to break the world record (put his mind and penis at ease by whispering, 'Don't hold back').

117 According to one survey, most men think women are not fond of the penis. Added to this are his insecurities about size and performance (see tip 109). So a woman who lets him know she likes his best friend is the equivalent of a man saying, **'You are the most wonderful woman I have ever met'.**

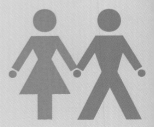

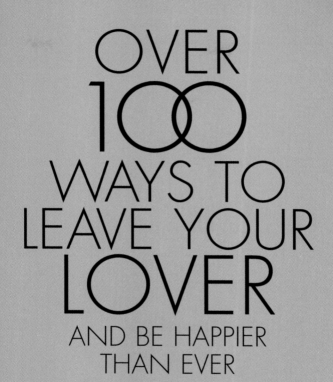

Section One

Denial

this isn't happening to me

Studies have found that it doesn't matter if you are the dumper or dumpee – EVERYONE has to go through emotional phases similar to grieving in order to deal with relationship meltdown.

The first stage is denial. As in, 'Huh? I didn't see it coming. OK, things haven't been working out for a while, but it's not like he's an axe murderer.'

The reality is, unless things are blatantly bad – he's hitting you, cheating on you with everything on the planet, wearing your clothes – it can be hard to be 100 per cent positive that this guy isn't your Mr Right. Even then, you may think, 'Maybe this is just a rough spot that we need to work through,' or, 'It's me – I'll change and things will get better.' Odds are, once you're feeling this way, they won't. Here's how to tell where to draw the line.

OVER AND OUT

Swift ways to figure out if he's the real deal
or if the two of you are history:

You're starting to **abhor** what you
used to **adore**. A University of Ohio
study found that there's a flip side
to love in that the things that first
attract us are often the very things
that start turning us off when the
relationship is skidding towards a
dead end. So his sexy take-charge
attitude now seems controlling. Your
fun-loving 'life of the party' suddenly
seems more like an odious flirt. And
his charming romantic streak begins
to feel needy and insecure.

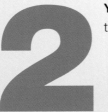

You argue over who started
the last big fight.

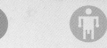

You're putting up with behaviour from him that you wouldn't normally tolerate from a bank teller or shoe salesman, let alone someone you supposedly love. Research by relationship guru Barbara De Angelis, PhD, has found that women – especially younger ones – are easily susceptible to the myth that **Love Conquers All** and will, therefore, stay in a relationship way past its prime in the hope that the man will (miraculously) change (see tips 15–19 for other bogus true romance beliefs).

Love him/Dump him

- You have good sex together regularly/ The only thing that's good about being together is the regular sex.
- He's yours/He's there.
- Looking at him, you think, 'How did I get so lucky?'/Looking at him, you wonder, 'WHAT was I thinking?'
- You know no-one will ever love you like he does/You fear no-one will ever ask you out again.
- His screensaver is a picture of you/His screensaver is a picture of a naked woman (not you).

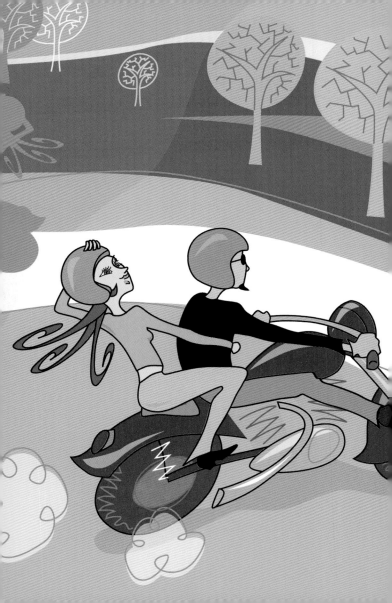

5 **A man from your past** shows up and, even though he's straight out of jail, you don't hesitate to straddle his Harley.

6 **You don't panic** that he may be flirting with his new assistant at work (the one you know for a fact is an ex-porn star).

7 **You hate** the way he breathes.

DON'T GET BURNED

Seven secret signs your man is about to bolt:

He's been criticizing you big time. According to communication experts, this is the typical male way of saying, 'I'm not really interested in you anymore,' while justifying his decision to bail. His secret wish? That you'll get so fed up, you'll say, 'I'm outta here.'

8

He introduces you as his **'friend'**.

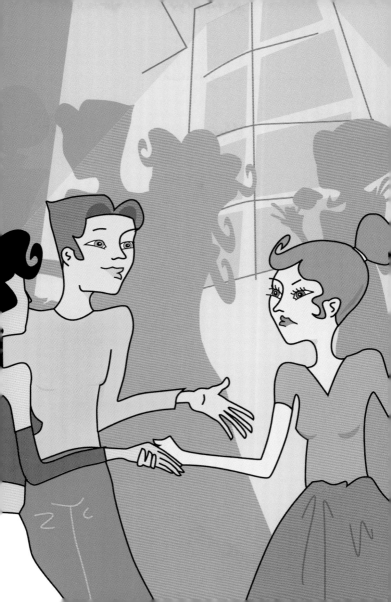

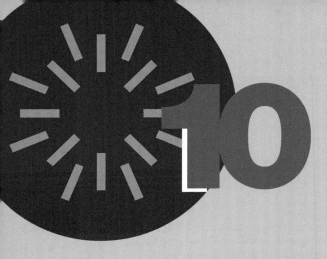

10

He asks you if you have ever thought about **having an affair** (translation: HE's thinking about it).

He suddenly starts making nice with you. According to a Texas Christian University study, there's a break-up blueprint that most people follow when they're getting ready to dissolve their partnership: you notice other people, you guiltily try to make things lovey-dovey with your own partner, you get pissed off with the effort, repeat the cycle twice and then call it quits.

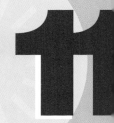

11

You notice a dramatic **shift in your sex life**. If you did it a lot, you now do it less, and vice versa. An Archives of Sexual Behaviour study discovered that the former happens because he's getting it elsewhere (or fantasizing about it); and the latter because he is desperately trying to make things work out.

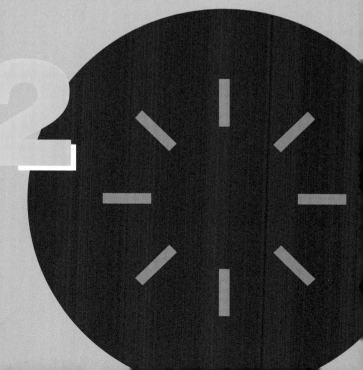

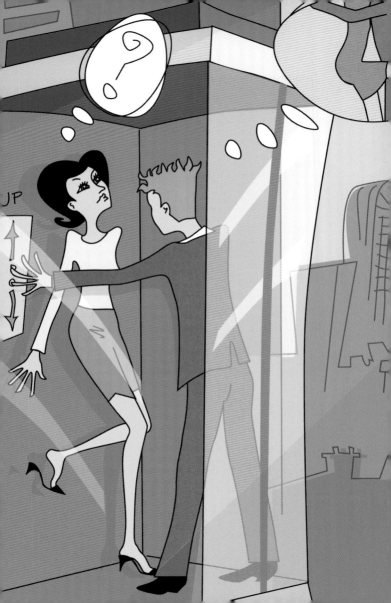

He suggests a repeat performance of that time you had amazing **sex in the lift** (elevator) – only you've never had sex in a lift.

He won't make plans for the future, even for tomorrow night. Research on men and communication confirms what you knew all along: guys are notorious for not breaking bad – or ANY – news. To avoid confrontation, he might stop talking, calling or e-mailing, or move to another city – anything to keep from telling you he wants out. If you do corner him, he's likely to stutter and stammer, make a joke out of it or blurt it out in a way that feels like a groin kick from Jackie Chan.

ONCE UPON A TIME

Unless you want to become the heartbreak queen, erase these love myths from your heart.

Myth: You think he is the only one.
Reality: Wrong. There are millions of potential soulmates for every person in the world.

Myth: Your heart will never fully recover.
Reality: It will.

Myth: True love conquers all.
Reality: True love doesn't conquer a lying, cheating bastard or even a Mr Not-Quite-Right who is perfectly sweet but leaves you yawning.

Myth: 'If only I were prettier, thinner or smarter (or whatever!), it would have worked out.'
Reality: You might be Gwyneth Paltrow's more gorgeous cousin who could kick ass on the *Weakest Link* and he'll still dump you if he wants out of the relationship.

8 19

Myth: When you have incredible body-melting sex with someone, it must be love.
Reality: When you have incredible body-melting sex with someone, it must be a great orgasm.

Section Two

Bargaining

should you let him go?

All you want to know is what you can do to **stop the pain. NOW**. You have reached stage two.

Obviously, it's always better to be the leaver than the leavee. First of all, because it's going to be more of an ego boost to be the one who is doing the dumping rather than the one who is getting dumped. But also, you need to be the one to call it a day if you think you might have even a remote interest in getting your ex back sometime in the future.

A slew of studies on the perverse workings of the human mind have found that we are more likely to want what we cannot have. Ergo: leave him and you instantly become catnip for him.

So here's how to let your man know that he is about to rejoin the singles world.

THE BLOW-OFF

A clean break is all in the timing.

AFTER A FEW DATES

THE METHOD: Become the invisible woman.

HOW TO DO IT: If you've just had one date, don't answer his calls or e-mails. He'll either (a) forget about you, (b) meet someone new or (c) assume you've been kidnapped by a cult. If you've had a few more dates but aren't really a 'relationship' yet, allow so much time to pass between dates that in the interim travel agents have started selling trips to Mars. Do this by screening your calls, hanging out where he doesn't and wearing a wig in public.

KEY PHRASES: If he happens to catch you unexpectedly, simply say you're so busy right now that you don't have time for anything but work. For the truly dense, you may have to use the 'I've met someone else' line (for other options, see tips 23 and 24).

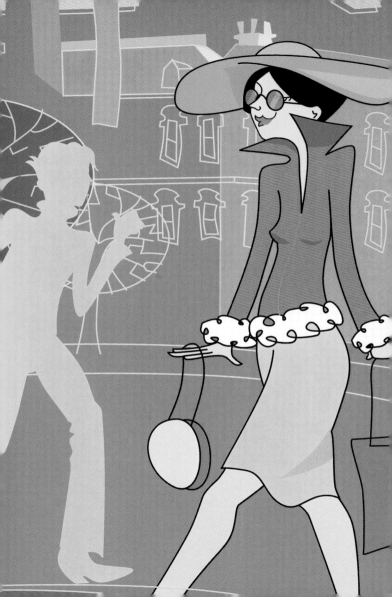

AFTER A FEW MONTHS

THE METHOD: Give him the old 'it's not you, it's me' speech. Polls show that although this is the least-used method, it's the most effective, as it keeps things from getting personal and therefore reduces the risk that he'll start hurling 'big ass' insults. That said, tip 28 also works well at this juncture.

HOW TO DO IT: Rehearse what you are going to say in advance. This will make it easier to keep to your script and not get sidetracked into unseemly 'discussions' about the size of his genitals (you) or your eerie similarity to your mother (him). Sit him down in a public place, such as a park (he's less likely to cry, beg or get violent). Avoid restaurants and pubs (he may retaliate to your dump method by dumping food or drink over your head).

21

KEY PHRASES: 'I'm not ready for commitment' or 'I want to concentrate on my career' are both hard for him to argue against. Another possibility: cite irreconcilable – and, if possible, irreversible – differences, such as his religion, profession, race, height and/or country of origin.

AFTER ONE OR MORE YEARS

THE METHOD: Draw it out (but not for so long that the break-up lasts longer than the relationship itself). This way, you work through your guilt, fears of being alone and the habit of the relationship before you actually spend a night as a newly single person.

> HOW TO DO IT: Have Discussions About The Relationship. Drop not-so-subtle hints about how you are losing interest. Talk about the things that really bug you (see suggestions under tip 28). Pick fights, then say, 'See? We're incompatible.' (Warning: this last one doesn't work with boyfriends in the mental health field – they'll simply call you passive-aggressive and hoodwink you into going to couples therapy.) Do this at 3 am when your defences are at their lowest.

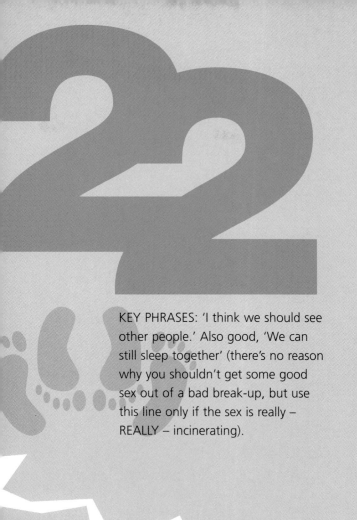

KEY PHRASES: 'I think we should see other people.' Also good, 'We can still sleep together' (there's no reason why you shouldn't get some good sex out of a bad break-up, but use this line only if the sex is really – REALLY – incinerating).

MAKE HIM SUFFER

According to research by Charles T Hill, PhD, of Whittier College, California, the quickest way to wound a guy where it hurts (read: his babe-magnet abilities) is to dump him.

LET HIM GO GENTLY: Butter him up with more flattery than he gets from his mother. Telling him he's a great person who will make someone very happy someday will make him feel so good he'll be eager to forget you and get on with wowing the rest of the female population.

PRICK HIM: Tell him you just want to be friends. Then offer to set him up with one of your friends, mentioning she hasn't been in a relationship for a while. He'll hear: (a) you see him as a sexless hang-out buddy, (b) who is not capable of getting his own dates and (c) is only fit for desperate women.

MAKE HIM CRY: Sleep with his best friend or brother. Remember that the best way to achieve a 'clean break' is to make it as harsh as possible, so the parties involved don't ever get to see each other again, partly due to sheer embarrassment and partly due to the restraining order.

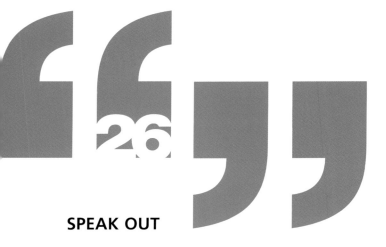

SPEAK OUT

Decipher his **favourite exit lines**:

'You're much too good for me.'
    Read: 'You're not the one.'
'I'm under a lot of pressure right now.'
    Read: 'I don't find you sexy any more.'
'I like you too much.'
    Read: 'I'm scared to get involved.'
'You're too together to put up with my crap.'
    Read: 'You're boring, I'm history.'
'I'm not ready to get serious.'
    Read: 'I am but not with you.'

If he has audacity to break up with you, sock it to him with these **survivor lines**:

'Phew. Now I don't have to confess about the affair I've been having.'

'Cool. I just met a hot guy and was wondering how to break it to you.'

'So now would not be a good time to tell you I've decided to become a lesbian?'

'Guess I won't be giving you that secret Eastern oral sex technique I learned as a surprise for your birthday.'

'Tell the truth – you're doing this because you feel bad that you've never been able to give me an orgasm, right?'

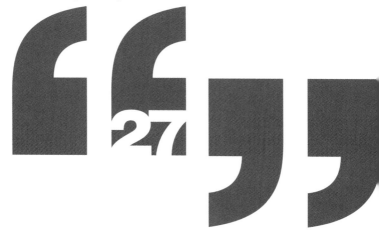

27

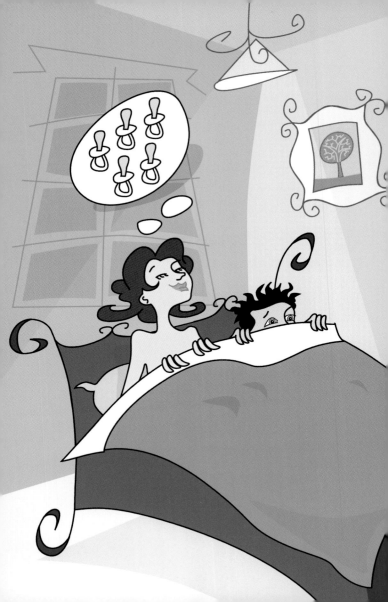

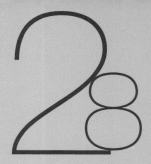

These **sneaky break-off tactics** are so devious, he'll think the break-up was HIS idea (poor fool).

- One night in bed, after a particularly hot-and-heavy session, murmur in his ear, 'I've always wanted five kids – what about you?'
- Pick, pick, pick on your soon-to-be ex-lover until he can't wait to leave.
- Become impossibly demanding, selfish and possessive until he loses all interest.
- Smother your partner with love – call him ten times a day, insist on spending every waking moment with him, and tell him he is your life. He'll be gone before you can say, 'You complete me.'
- Tell him that you have decided to become a born-again virgin and plan to hold off on sex until you get married.
- Get caught with your pants down (see tip 25, Make Him Cry).

BREAKING UP IS HARD TO DO

If you're too chicken to say the words yourself, try one of these ready-made aids.

Send a card that 'bulls-eyes' your I-love-you-not message. Simply handwrite a personalized message and on-line greeting card company **www.sparks.com** will send it for you via regular old snail mail or e-mail. For those who prefer the cut-and-dried method, try this message: 'Although our lives have only crossed each other's paths for a short period of time, I can already tell you this … it's been long enough.'

When you want to avoid that I-wish-I-said-that feeling, log onto the Cyrano website at **www.nando.net/toys/cyrano.html** They'll write a personalized goodbye for you based on information you type in. Easy-peasy.

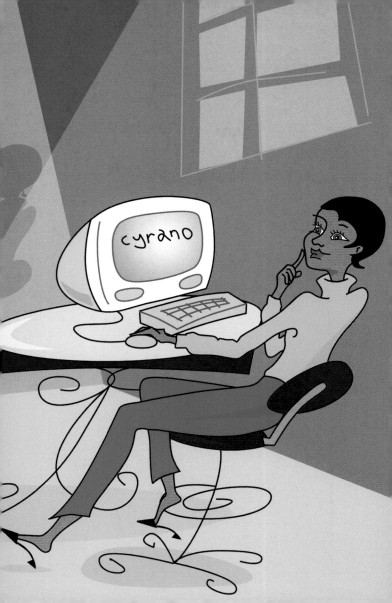

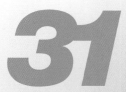

31

If the indirect approach is more your style, send an **anonymous note** and a trial-size bug repellent through the post, direct to his door.

If Romeo needs things spelled out more clearly, visit **www.dfilm.com**, where you can single-handedly produce a digital, animated short staging your break-up scenario, complete with soundtrack.

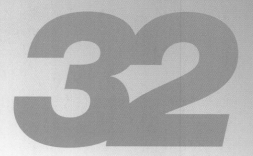

32

Tell your boyfriend **you have to talk**. Then put on Paul Simon's 'Fifty Ways To Leave Your Lover', Carol King's 'It's Too Late' or Nancy Sinatra's 'These Boots Were Made For Walking' and walk out the door.

33

Say, **'You'll be needing this'** and give him one of Melissa Etheridge's early CDs.

34

Section Three

Depression

I can't believe this is
happening to me

You've just entered Splitsville (population: you). And it hurts bad, even if you were the one who downsized him.

That's because breaking up is more than just saying goodbye. It's easy to delete his number from your speed dial; it's a lot harder to get him out of your heart. Researchers at the Medical College of Virginia have found that no matter who dumped who, your likelihood of depression rises 1,130 per cent after the end up of a relationship. Hello, stage three!

Bottom line: recovery isn't going to happen overnight. Truly getting over someone takes effort. Here's your plan for getting him off your mind – and having a little fun at the same time.

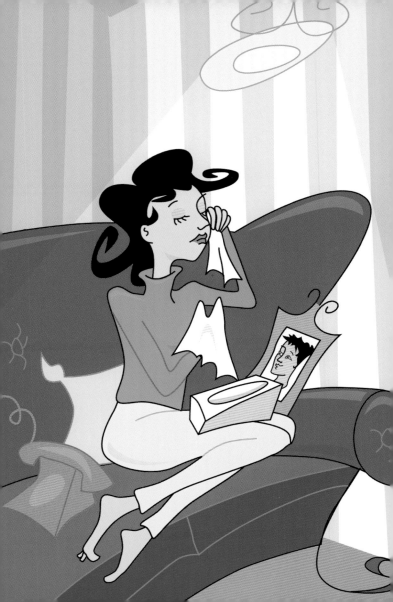

TOTAL REBOUND

Follow this guide to help you dry your tears, lighten your heart and survive the first 24 hours.

35 All you want to do is **sit alone** on the floor with a candle burning and Toni Braxton wailing 'You Break My Heart' on the stereo. So go ahead – brood over him, linger over every detail of the relationship. Many people ignore or deny their pain, pretending they're doing fine. Big mistake. Psychologists have found that you need to give in to your misery now, so the feelings don't drag on and on and invade every future relationship you have with other guys, with your friends, or even with yourself (see tips 39 and 52 if you need help getting in the mood).

36 **Weep**. Snivel. Blubber. According to an Oklahoma University Health Science Center study, crying lowers blood pressure and relaxes muscles, making it a great natural tranquilliser for reducing physical and emotional agitation. But only if you tell someone about your sorrow as soon as your tears have dried (see tips 64–71 for who to call).

Take heart: the more you hurt, the better a person you are. One study found that it's the truly 'good' people – trusting, vulnerable and loving souls – who are the ones that really hurt when a relationship ends. Another upside – these are also the people who get a lot more out of life than the people who claim they've never had their heart broken.

Take out your calendar and **choose a date** to end the pity party and pull yourself together. Research has confirmed that you need to set a deadline to your emotional torment before getting on with repairing your heart (skip down to the Fix Your Heart – Fast section, tips 45–76, for some quick remedies).

Take the **sad song** cure. Play Sade, The Smiths, Alanis Morissette – any music that gives the illusion that the whole world understands how you feel right now.

As for 'your song', **avoid sobbing** whenever you hear it by giving the song a new memory. Play the song with some good friends and dance on tables, stand on your heads – do anything that will make you burst out laughing the next time you hear it.

Throw an Ex Party. Rule out anyone handing out 'you'd feel better if you got out of bed' advice (you won't). You want sympathetic souls who will listen to you endlessly recount every detail of the break-up. Let them dole out tissues and cookies, tell you you're right, that you're not getting stress zits, remind you that you're a totally smart, fab babe and give you shoulder rubs (all that tension from crying!).

Don't call him. No ifs, ands or buts. Even if you broke up with him. If he calls you, don't pick up. Studies have found you need at least a one-week breather before sane talk is even possible.

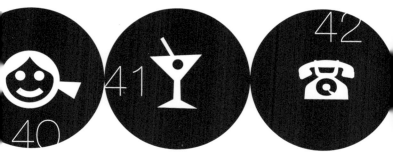

43

Use cucumber slices or cold teabags to reduce the puffiness around your eyes. Drink lots of water – it will make you feel less dehydrated after crying.

44

Do not – **DO NOT** – phone him. Especially after drinking five Cosmopolitans. Set all your speed dials to your best friend so if you do try and call him, you'll end up ringing her (she can then remind you that it's over and you are way too good for him).

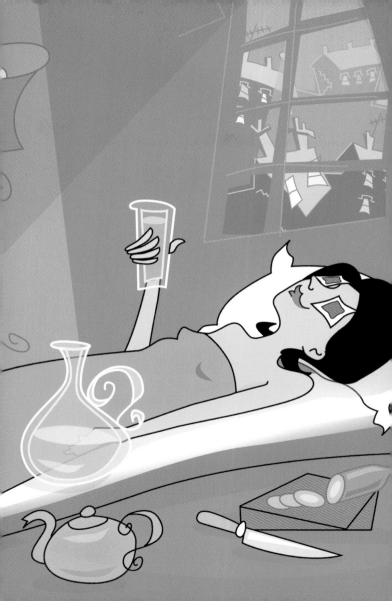

FIX YOUR HEART – FAST

Follow these tips to learn how to bounce back and jump-start your life (and heart) again.

Focus on today. Take things one step at a time, one day at a time. Relationship experts say that if you start looking towards or thinking about next week, next month or next year, you'll feel overwhelmed.

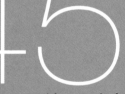

Set aside a period of time each day for grieving. You're allowed to wallow in self-pity between, say, 7 and 7:30 every evening. If you find yourself thinking about HIM at 9:13 am, tell yourself you'll think about that during the allotted time.

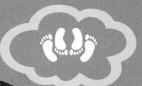

Don't lie in bed all day fantasizing about
the last great orgasm you had with him.

47

Adopt a pet. Experts say that interacting with pets can reduce blood pressure, increase the rate of healing and ease depression. Pet therapists use animals to help alleviate these symptoms among critically ill patients, and there's no reason why you can't get the same benefits (if it was a nasty break-up, adopt a pit bull terrier and take him for frequent walks around your ex's block).

Give yourself a pinch for every negative 'No-one will ever love me again' thought. This process is called retraining your brain. Ouch.

Give yourself one week to indulge – eat nothing, eat just Ben and Jerry's, go out and party, go on a shopping spree (with HIS credit cards), flirt with the postman, have (protected) meaningless sex. Then stop and reassess. Studies show this cooling-off period will help give you distance and perspective.

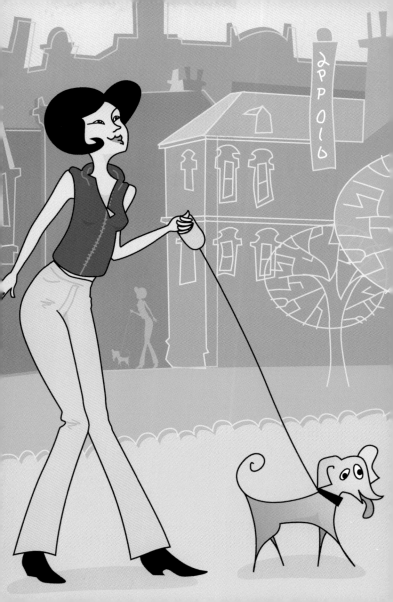

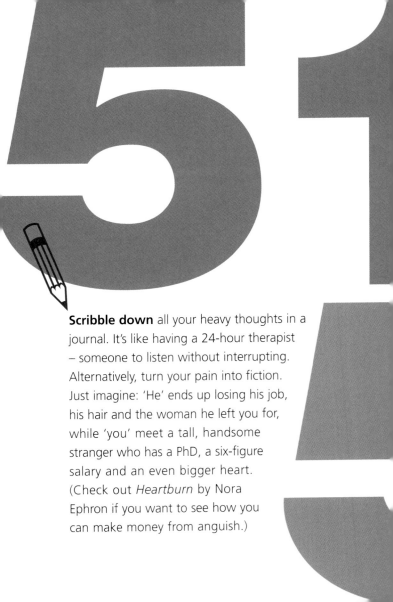

Scribble down all your heavy thoughts in a
journal. It's like having a 24-hour therapist
– someone to listen without interrupting.
Alternatively, turn your pain into fiction.
Just imagine: 'He' ends up losing his job,
his hair and the woman he left you for,
while 'you' meet a tall, handsome
stranger who has a PhD, a six-figure
salary and an even bigger heart.
(Check out *Heartburn* by Nora
Ephron if you want to see how you
can make money from anguish.)

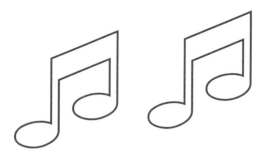

Put your pain in perspective. Listen to country music or watch a daytime talk show (in your current state of mind, you'll be able to totally relate).

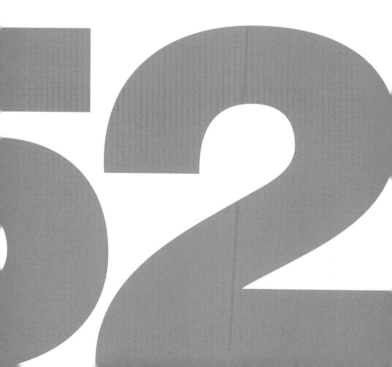

53

Go on a chocolate diet. Chocolate contains a natural amphetamine, phenylethylamine, the same one our brains produce when we fall in love and that makes us feel giddy and elated. When we fall out of love, we have PEA withdrawal.

Just Do It. You probably don't much feel like breaking a sweat, but research shows that working out for just 30 minutes a day is a major mood-buster (and gut-buster if you've been following tip 53). Your body starts pumping out endorphins, those all-natural feel-good chemicals which not only kill your pain, but also make you feel inspired, strong and chock-full of self-confidence (plus you'll look fabulous if you run into him again). The added bonus: pretend the ball you're hitting, the punchbag you're slugging or the pavement you're pounding is his face.

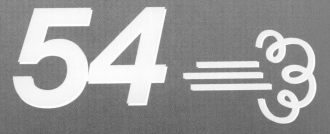

54

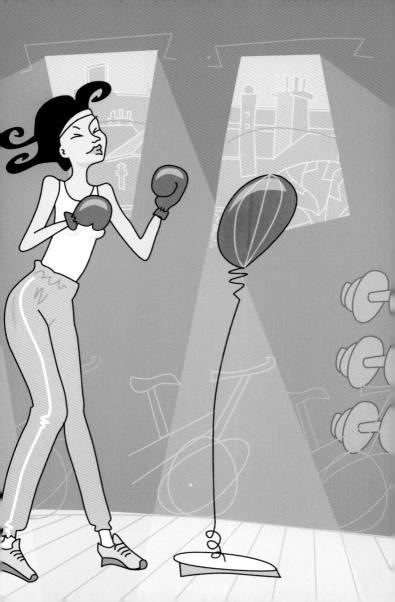

Put a **positive spin** on what is happening. You may feel rejected and a failure because your relationship has disintegrated, but for every drawback there is an advantage. Don't think of it as a 'failure', but a 'transition'. You aren't 'abandoned' or 'left behind', you are 'ready for something new'. Write down all the negative statements that occur to you, and then rewrite every single one of them with a positive slant.

Call up an old friend who used to have a big-time crush on you for a little confidence-booster.

Weekends are tough for the newly single woman. Form a Saturday Night Club and have a standing date with a bunch of similarly solo friends.

Reprogram your thoughts. Stop mid-sentence if you've been obsessing about what you could have/should have/would have done differently. Instead, change your chant to what you can't/won't/shouldn't ever do or take in a relationship again. The point? When you check out what happened or what went wrong in a relationship, you can figure out how to try to make sure it doesn't go wrong again, or if it does, to at least (hopefully) recognize it when it's happening (or, you can just blame him).

Give yourself six weeks. According to studies, this is about how long it takes to get over a severe loss.

Vow NOT to swear off men. Research has found women who avoid any emotional attachment after a bad break-up are much more likely to leave or destroy their next relationship for fear of getting hurt again.

Wait at least **90 days** before having sex again (think of it as your ex-relationship's warranty). Apparently, researchers have found that this is enough time to let your body get charged up for sex again.

Send his stuff packing. Studies show that we get physically addicted to the pheromones secreted by the person we sleep with. So by cleaning the house, you're psychologically telling yourself that you are making room for something (or someone!) new.

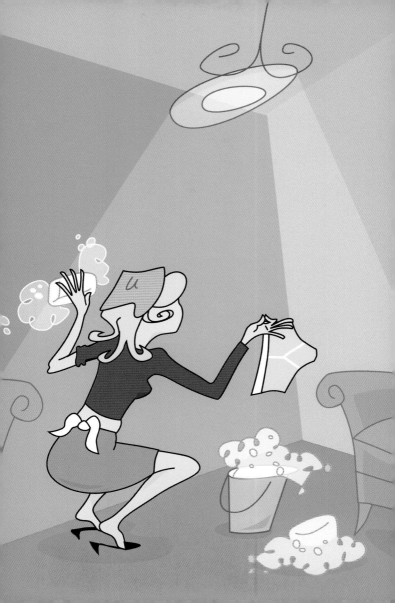

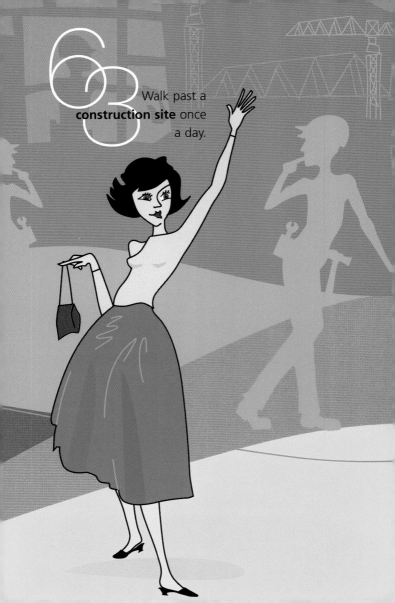

63

Walk past a
construction site once
a day.

SOCIAL RUTS

Match your mood to your support system.

64

Visit your mother if you want to be babied and cooked your favourite foods.

Find your dad if you just want to hang out silently with someone and maybe hammer a few things.

35

66

Call your best friend when you need to hear how sexy, smart and wonderful you are.

Get together with a happily married couple if you need instant proof that being back with the 'singletons' is better.

67

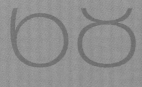

68 Gather single girlfriends when you're ready to go prowling for fresh meat and **have catty bitch sessions** about your ex (they've been there, done it and bought the T-shirt).

69 **Dial male friends** when you need reminding that not all men are swine.

70 Look up **an old ex** for a passionate fling.

71 **Get in touch with his friends** when you need to let out all the venomous things you have ever felt about him. It should (a) get back to your ex and (b) allow you to gauge whether the listener likes or dislikes your ex, perhaps giving you something in common in case you wish to shoot for tip 25 with any of them.

EX HIM OUT

Exorcise your ex for good.

72

Go ahead and give in to your impulse to gab about him 24/7. A group of students at the University of Virginia were told to talk for ten minutes about any topic EXCEPT an old flame. After, when asked to think about their exes, their bodies showed high stress. Conclusion: you NEED to verbally agonize in order to heal.

Instead of seeing him as **Ex-Guy Love God**, change your mental image to Ex-Guy Anal Retentive, a mental, midget, control freak, who loses it if you have to work even an hour late.

73

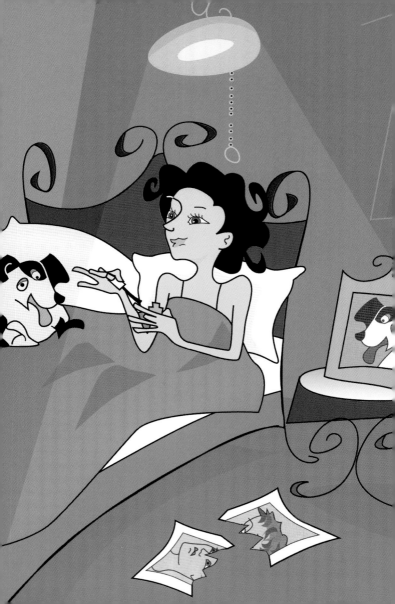

Replace the photograph of him next to your bed with one of your precious pooch.

Make a list – yes one of THOSE – about everything that was bad about the relationship (be honest!). He nagged you. You didn't trust him. You didn't have a lot in common. You get the picture. Carry the list for the next few days to get you over the 'I want him back' hump. Refer to it as necessary.

Insert **'bastard'** (or some similar epitaph) every time you say or think his name.

Section Three

Anger

why does this have
to happen to me?

This is the 'Arrgh! I'm so mad I could spit' stage. Bitterness and regret rule as you obsess how you gave this man three good dates/months/years – time that could have been spent doing … well, other things. With other men! You're not sure with whom, but they would have been awesome. Instead, you were working like a dog to build something real and lasting with that (fill in appropriate noun). Well, if he thinks he can treat you like that, forget about it.

The thing about anger is that you need it for recovery – experts have found that a little outrage goes a long way towards stimulating adrenaline, making you feel stronger and more confident. The danger is that you can get so stuck in your 'he loses his hair/job/life' fantasies that you don't move on with your own life.

Don't fight your rage; feel the pain, but direct it. Here's how to get mad, get even and then get over him.

REVENGE IS SWEET

Make him pay without risk.

77

You may think you need to **trash him** to move on. But according to research, getting revenge is exactly what prevents you from moving on. Apparently, every second you waste focused on him is one second less that you are going to feel better. If you can't help yourself, see tips 80, 81 and 83 for how to do it without leaving a trace.

78

Write a hate letter to your ex. Then destroy it. Repeat as often as necessary.

79

Get together with your friends and, using a doll, hold a mock funeral for him. Or destroy his photo, slowly ripping it as if you were tearing out his heart.

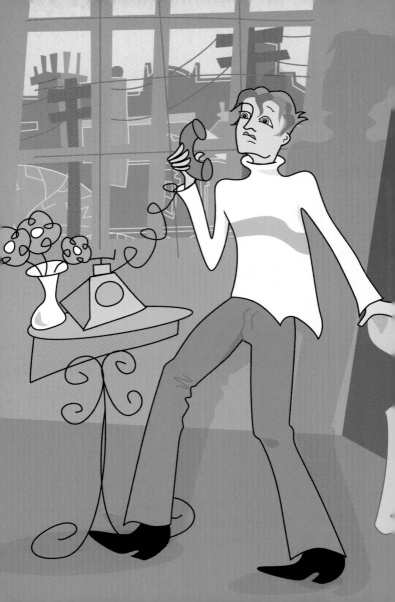

80

If you must get him, **keep it legal**. Call and tell him you have an STD (this is a double whammy because he'll think you were cheating on him). Get him a personal ad, saying he prefers 'full-bodied,' older women. Report all his credit cards as stolen. Sign him up for every piece of free junk e-mail under the sun. If he doesn't change his phone security code (and who ever does?), check his messages and delete any important ones (translation: those from women and bosses).

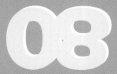

Check out these ultimate revenge websites; they'll do all your evil work for you:

www.virtual-design.com/demos/voodoodoll
Design your own virtual voodoo doll to torture and e-mail him the gruesome playback.
www.flwyd.dhs.org/curse When you've run out of every four-letter word in your vocabulary, pick one from the Elizabethan Curse Generator.
www.anonymizer.com Send all the vicious stuff you want and NEVER get traced or found out.
www.dogdoo.com Get down and dirty and send him virtual doggie poo.
www.deathclock.com For true peace of mind you can find out when your ex's time on earth is up.

81

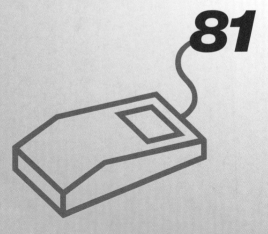

82

Plan your revenge in detail. Psychologists say that, for example, dreaming that you called his boss about him skimming money on his accounts so he gets fired without a reference, never gets another job, ends up homeless and alone, etc., is better than actually doing it. It reminds you that you have the power, girl. You just choose to use it only for good.

83

Use your pain and get creative. Alanis Morissette hit it big with her Grammy-winning song 'You Oughta Know' about getting dumped; Carly Simon grossed $2.5 million from her song about a vain ex-lover; Ivana Trump has made millions playing the trump card after The Donald left her for a younger model; and Mia Farrow received $3 million for trashing her life with Woody Allen, after he left her for her adopted daughter.

84

Know your local revenge laws; it could serve you well. In Singapore, a 32-year-old woman who made more than 60 crank calls a day to her ex's fiancée was fined almost £5,000 for harassment.

EX-FILES

Your manual for surviving sickeningly common close ex-encounters (no tissues required).

THE SITUATION: Arranging to return each other's personal stuff after the split.

DO: Make a list of everything that's yours and tell him he can do the same. If you don't think you can maintain your cool, get a friend to do the drop-off for you. Alternatively, arrange a blind drop-off in front of each other's homes.

DON'T: Meet at venues where you're likely to be flooded with nostalgic 'wasn't it wonderful' memories and either fall into a weeping heap or a sizzling snog for the trade-off. Also, don't bother with anything that's not valuable or has no sentimental value – replace it with a newer, better one.

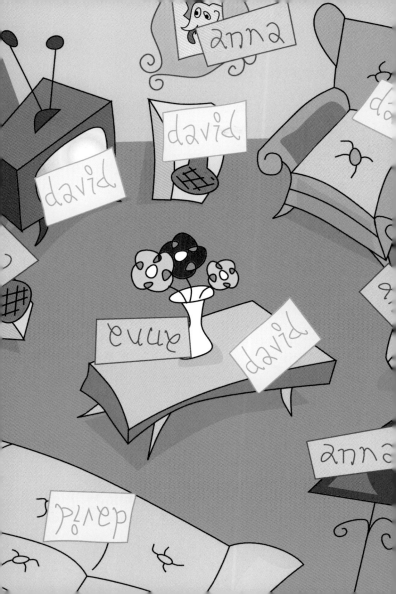

THE SITUATION: The first post-break-up encounter.

86

DO: Accept that you're probably going to hate how you look, even if you look fabulous. Let HIM say the first sentence after the initial greetings. Then casually say you'd love to talk (this is key – otherwise it looks like you are avoiding him), but you have to meet someone. Saunter off straight to the nearest phone to call your closest friend, telling her in detail what he was wearing, what he said, how he said it, etc.

DON'T: Start crying, laughing hysterically, talking non-stop or mauling him.

SITUATION: Seeing him talking (or flirting!) with another woman.

DO: Give him a teensy smile (as in, 'Uh-huh, got your number, dude'), nod and walk, don't run, straight to the nearest phone ... you know the drill.

DON'T: Approach him, find your own boy model to flirt with or collapse in a soppy, snivelling mess.

SITUATION: Meeting at a party and, 'accidentally' getting together.

DO: Accept that it happens. A lot. So don't dwell on it.

DON'T: Call him. What can you say to him that hasn't been said already? Think of it as your goodbye 'kiss'.

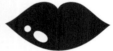

SITUATION: Bumping into him and his pretty new girlfriend.

DO: Smile. Be civil. Ask how he's doing. Say hi to the new babe. Then find that best friend. Unless, of course, you're with YOUR new guy. Who happens to look exactly like George Clooney (dream come true!). In which case, flaunt it.

DON'T: Be tempted to spill all the gory moments of your break-up to your new guy or his new girl. If either ask, just say, 'We used to go out.'

9 USES FOR AN EX-BOYFRIEND

Your relationship wasn't a total waste of time.

Comeback to your mum
When she gives her 'Why aren't you married like all your sisters and cousins' speech, simply say, 'Well you didn't want me to marry that last loser, did you?'

Wake-up call
Keep a picture of your ex to remind yourself that you should be dating men who didn't skip a link in the evolutionary chain.

Exercise incentive
You'd rather detour miles than risk running into him on his old turf.

Blame magnet
Make him the scapegoat for everything bad in your life – the backpack you can't find, the bad mood you're in, your addiction to KitKats.

Urge to splurge
Now you have the perfect excuse to toss out those old faded sheets.

95

Stress relief
Smash anything
he left behind to
smithereens.

Artistic inspiration
For your soon-to-be
critically acclaimed
work, entitled
'Ex Out'.

96

Wild sex

97

Getting smarter
Relationship psychologists say the best
thing an ex is good for is to figure out what
traits you DON'T want in a boyfriend.

98

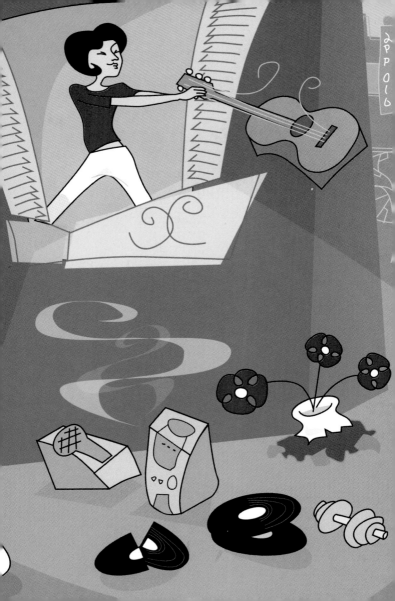

Section Five

Acceptance

it happened and I'll live
to love again

OK, you're through to the final lap. You have acknowledged the plain fact that the relationship is over ('Whew, it's been six weeks since we ended it and I realized the other day I haven't thought about him for one whole day').

Most psychologists agree that during this process you learn to accept yourself and become ready to move on. You've vented your feelings, now it is time to go beyond merely surviving the heartbreak and figuring out how to avoid it in the future.

This means:
(1) Keeping a level head when it comes to dating;
(2) taking an emotional inventory so you know what you want and expect out of your next relationship (quick fling versus real thing); and,
(3) most importantly, having faith – even if you are a vile wicked witch, there is an equally vile warlock out there for you.

WRAP IT UP

You're finally over him when …

You genuinely hope he is happy when you hear he's with someone new.

You can go to what used to be your **favourite restaurant**, eat what used to be your favourite dish AND enjoy it.

He calls, saying he made a **big mistake** and wants you to come back, and you put him on hold to take a call from your mother.

You finally toss out all the love mementos – not because they cause you pain, but because you need the shelf space.

You compare **New Guy to Ex-Guy** and instead of thinking New Guy comes up short, you realize New Guy is a total upgrade from Ex-Guy ('Wow! Ex-Guy never gave me an hour-long back massage.' 'Huh! Ex-Guy never listened when I complained about work.' 'Mmm. Ex-Guy could never find my G-Spot.').

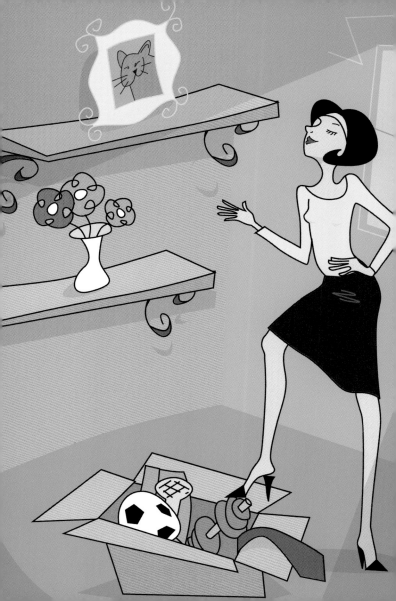

SINGLED OUT

Why it's great to be single (honest).

You can **flirt** with your (incredibly cute) local bartender without your guy shooting green laser beams into your back.

104

You don't have to **hang out** with your ex's slacker friend anymore (the one who thought playing air guitar was a talent).

105

You can spend the night drooling over **Brad Pitt** flicks without hearing a lot of snide remarks.

107

You can swap Rush Hour 2-meets-American Pie movies for **chick flicks without guilt**.

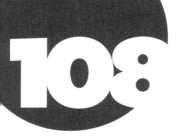

108 Did we mention **flirting** with your (incredibly cute) local bartender?

109 When you **have sex** with someone new, he doesn't wonder why you no longer want to do that kinky little thing he likes so much.

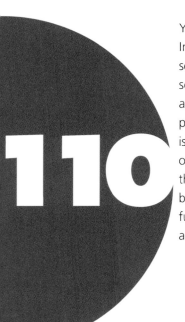

110 You get precious **alone-time**. In researching the effects of sensory deprivation, the ultimate solitude, Peter Suedfeld, PhD, a University of British Columbia psychologist who studies isolation, found that after just one hour of being totally on their own, people show lower blood pressure, higher mental functioning, enhanced creativity and a more positive outlook.

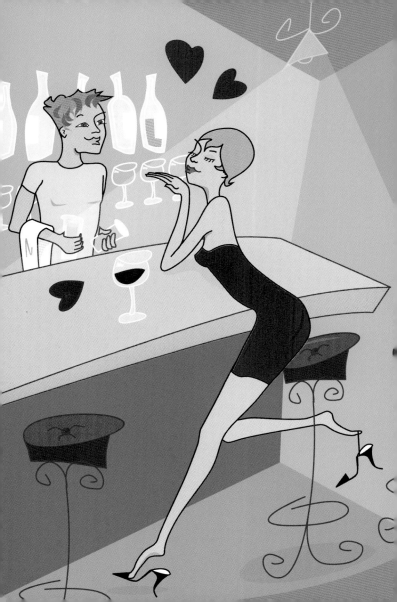

LOVER, COME BACK

Do you really want him back?

111 **Take two or three weeks to think** about restarting the connection. Suddenly being alone can feel terrible and alienating, and a lot of people have the knee-jerk reaction of wanting to make the loneliness go away by getting the other person back.

112 **Which of the following** thought processes best describes your current reality?
(a) It's not like I'm home every night sighing over him. It's been more than two weeks since we broke up. But I still dig him. And I can see where things went wrong and how we can work it out this time.
(b) Getting back together with my ex is better than being miserable and alone.
(c) I'm planning to dump his sorry ass the minute he takes me back.

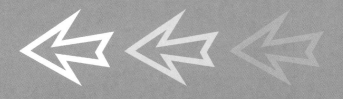

It's (a) or nothing. Psychologists say if you have a life without your ex, but you've been thinking about your relationship and have realized that, uh, actually you still like him, you're thinking clearly. Ergo: your chances of staying together second time around are good. Any other answer means that you're still hurting. Get back together with him now, and you may never recover. And you'll probably kill a good deal of self-esteem as well.

3 If tip 112 holds true for you, then **go for it**. When Nancy Kalish, PhD, studied more than 500 couples that had called it quits, she found a surprising 72 per cent reunited and stayed together. The reason? They now had more realistic expectations of what they both wanted out of the relationship.

4 **But wait at least a year**. In the same study, Dr Kalish found that the longer a couple stayed apart, the more successful their reunion. Seems you need time to carve out your own identity and not be so-and-so's girlfriend for a while before you can truly decide if you WANT to be his arm jewellery again.

LOVE TURNAROUND

Caution: If he dumped you and is now creeping back, his reasons are not necessarily honourable.

He misses the sex. Hey, he's a man and he has needs! He wants his usual and customary style of loving with a partner he is familiar with. He feels safe with you and comfortable, because you know what he likes. But sex is not enough to keep a man – never has been and never will be. Things will deteriorate right back to square one because he is not there for the long haul, only a quick roll.

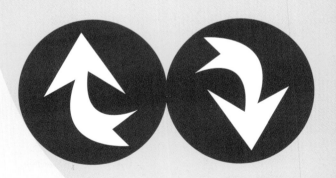

He needs to know you still care. In other words, he has seen you out on the town having a good time with some hot dude and needs to know he hasn't been replaced. His goal is to stay in contact with you and maintain your focus on him, just enough to keep the door open IN CASE he decides later that he wants to come back to you.

He doesn't want to start over. Thinking about the time he will need to spend trying to replace you is overwhelming. He thinks about the energy required to establish a foundation and framework for a new relationship and he gets a headache. He would rather apologize, give you what you want and just move on down the road with the woman who understands him and shares a history with him. Basically, he is lazy and would rather fight than switch.

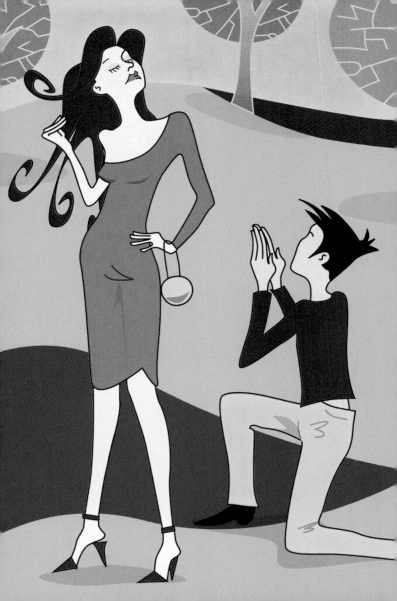

He realizes he messed up bad. He has a chronic case of guilt. Now that he has had time away from you and the situation, he's come to the shocking realization that he truly cares for you (more than he knew). Don't keel over, it may be the dreaded 'L' word at work here! He has gone out, dated other women, hung out with his guy friends, and realized he isn't having the big fun he thought he would. His life is empty and meaningless without you in it. He is depressed, unmotivated, moody and very unhappy. He comes to you to get back together when he is willing to make the adjustments and apologies and changes needed to return the relationship to its former level of focus and commitment, and move forward in love. To demonstrate his seriousness, he may make promises of a future and offer homes, cars, trips *and* wedding rings. In short, go for it.

HAPPILY EVER AFTER

Your checklist for figuring out if it's time to get back in the love saddle.

119 If you **think about your ex at least once a day** (or are still having sex with him), would take your ex back in a heartbeat (even if you were dating someone else), have a crush on a man because he reminds you of your ex, still carry your ex's photo or feel like you are never going to be in love again, then you are in no way ready to jump-start your love life. Psychologists warn that if you starting to date before you've recovered from your old relationship, you could set up a situation where you man-hop in your search for eternal love. To stop the madness, do the drill in tip 58. Only when you understand what went wrong in the last relationship can you figure out how to avoid it again.

120 **Consider your motives** for wanting to date again. A love affair is not a cure-all for what ails you. Polls have found that the people who are happiest being in a relationship are the ones who are also happiest being on their own (see tip 110).

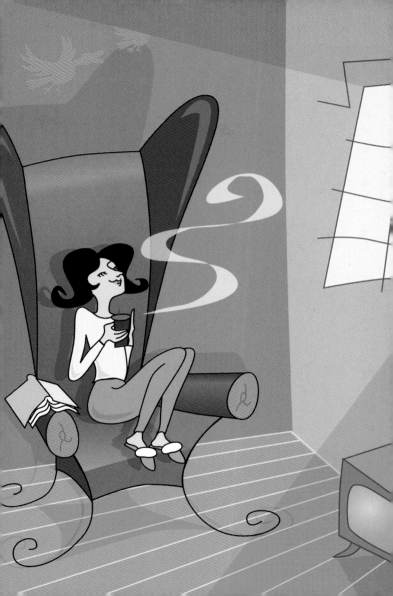

You are ready for new love when you can deal with **answering questions** about your last relationship without auto-crying, blaming him or ranting.

Bouncing back into a **new romance** can be a good cure for a broken heart. It dulls the pain, numbs the loss and revives your shattered self-esteem, but only if you slip into it with the right attitude. You should want to have fun, not a relationship.

Repeatedly ask yourself: **Would I want this guy for a friend?** Studies have found that the best post-break-up boyfriend is a man who reminds you of your male friends rather than of your ex. These are the guys you've always enjoyed hanging out with on a Saturday afternoon and whose values you share.